Nina Barough

WALKING
FOR FITNESS

Nina Barough

WALKING FOR FITNESS

Penguin
Random
House

To all those who put their trust in me and Walked the Walk

This edition
US Development Editor Kayla Dugger
US Managing Editor Lori Hand
Senior Editor Kate Meeker
Design Assistant Philippa Nash
Jacket Designer Steve Marsden
Pre-Production Manager Sunil Sharma
Senior DTP Designer Pushpak Tyagi
Pre-producer Robert Dunn
Producer Olivia Jeffries
Managing Editor Stephanie Farrow
Managing Art Editor Christine Keilty
US Publisher Mike Sanders

Original edition
Project Editor Jennifer Lane
Art Editor Ruth Hope
Senior Editor Jennifer Jones
Managing Editor Gillian Roberts
Managing Art Editor Karen Sawyer
Category Publisher Mary-Clare Jerram
DTP Designer Sonia Charbonnier

First American Edition, 2003
This edition published in the United States in 2017 by
DK Publishing, 345 Hudson Street, New York, New York 10014

A catalog record for this book
is available from the Library of Congress.
ISBN 978-1-4654-5888-9

DK books are available at special discounts when purchased
in bulk for sales promotions, premiums, fund-raising, or
educational use. For details, contact: DK Publishing Special
Markets, 345 Hudson Street, New York, New York 10014
SpecialSales@dk.com

Printed and bound in China

All images © Dorling Kindersley Limited
For further information see:
www.dkimages.com

A WORLD OF IDEAS:
SEE ALL THERE IS TO KNOW
www.dk.com

CONTENTS

AUTHOR'S FOREWORD

This is a book about discovering how to power walk and the astounding number of benefits that come with it. It is about not only learning how our bodies work, but also realizing that our attitudes and beliefs, what we eat and drink, and even how we breathe all create who we are. You will find out how small and simple changes can ultimately have a huge impact on your health, fitness, and quality of life.

In 1997 I discovered I had breast cancer. My world fell apart, and all the beliefs and ideals that I had held for so many years were suddenly challenged and put to the absolute test. I am not sure whether I supported the charity Walk the Walk I had started only months earlier or it supported me, but what I do know is that I became totally focused on my health, and this is when the wonders of power walking really became apparent to me.

During my months of treatment, I used power walking, diet, vitamins, positive thinking, and visualization to help manage and conquer my cancer, and as a result I became fitter, had more energy, and felt more vibrant and balanced than at any other time in my life.

For me, walking is magical. After a few minutes I start to feel my shoulders relax, my chest open, my breath begins to deepen, and my lungs fill with air. Best of all, I feel as though I have shaken off a heavy cloak, and the day's activities fall away from me. After 30 minutes of powerful walking, nothing ever seems that big or bad, and I feel great. It is my biggest wish that this book will not only encourage you to step out of your door and start walking, but inspire you to look at all aspects of your life.

Enjoy your walking!

THE POWER OF WALKING

We all have dreams of becoming fitter, leaner, and stronger, and bursting with health and energy. Power walking can bring you all these benefits. The technique provides a simple yet effective way of giving your whole body a thorough workout. You may also discover, as many others have, that power walking opens you up to new experiences, and that it brings mental well-being as well as physical health.

"Twenty years from now you will be more disappointed by the things you didn't do than by the ones you did. So throw off the bowlines. Sail away from the safe harbor. Catch the trade winds in your sails. Explore. Dream. Discover." MARK TWAIN

WHAT IS POWER WALKING?

Walking is the most natural and fundamental of all human conscious movements; by putting one foot in front of the other and moving your arms in opposition, you can propel yourself forward at approximately 3 mph (5km/h). Add the "power," change your focus, adjust your technique, and the pace can increase to 5 mph (8km/h) or more. All the muscles in your body are used to create a dynamic aerobic activity that helps you to achieve optimum well-being and fitness.

Many people take up walking as a hobby or for the sake of fitness because it is so accessible. It is a low-impact form of exercise because it does not put undue stress and strain on your joints. This means it carries a low risk of injury. You also don't need to go through the pain threshold as you do with some other sports; it is up to you to choose how challenging you want it to be.

Categories of walking

There are five main walking styles, though they come with a confusing variety of titles—for example, athletic walking, fitness walking, and dynamic walking are all names used for power walking. However, the five categories are quite clearly defined by speed and technique.

The stroll This is a casual pace, slower than the average walk. A person strolling would find that it takes around 30 minutes or more to walk a mile (20 minutes or more to walk a kilometer).

THE POPULAR CHOICE

Walking used to be considered an easy option in exercise, or as nothing more than a way of getting from A to B. Walking for health and fitness is now a highly popular sport for all ages, with millions of people taking part worldwide, on their own or in groups. Power or fitness walking has gained such popularity that it is now a more common route to fitness than running.

The average walk Everyone has their own walking speed in everyday life, but the average is considered to be approximately 3 mph (5km/h). This would mean an average walker would take 20 minutes to walk a mile (12 minutes to walk a kilometer), though most people probably could not sustain this speed for more than an hour or so.

Power walking The stroll and the average walk are defined simply by speed because technique is not much of a consideration. You will naturally swing your arms in opposition to your legs to aid your balance and to help you to move forward. However, with the next pace, power walking, the technique is specific and important.

A power walker can reach speeds of up to 5 mph (8km/h), which means walking a mile in 12 minutes (a kilometer in less than 8 minutes). To propel forwards, a power walker pushes off each stride from the toes with a straight back leg for extra strength and stability. This is where the power comes from and why the push-off is so important. The arm movement is also vital to a power walker's speed and drive, with both elbows at a 90-degree angle, arms punching back and forth in a pistonlike action. Turn to pp42–49 to read about the technique.

Speed walking This is the next category as you step up your exertion a gear from power walking. The pace of a speed walker is in excess of 5 mph (8km/h). A useful description of speed walking is to think that it is in relation to racewalking as jogging is to running. A power walker who continually works at his or her speed will eventually reach this category naturally.

Racewalking Also known as Olympic walking, this is the ultimate pace with regard to speed. Racewalkers reach speeds of 9 mph (14.5km/h) or more, and are mainly concerned with speed and competing (*see pp106–107 for more information on the rules*). They have their own technique and strict rules and move with the familiar hip-roll and wiggle that many people think of when power walking is mentioned. The technique used for power walking is a simplified forerunner of racewalking.

Perfecting the pace

The beauty of power walking is that you can progress from being an average walker to a power walker in a matter of weeks. Putting in the extra effort to begin power walking, rather than just

Power walkers always give the impression that they are striding along with great purpose and determination, which they most probably are.

strolling, means that your heart rate will be raised to a higher level. Working the heart in this way is what makes power walking a cardiovascular aerobic activity that is perfect for keeping you fit and healthy (*see pp34–35*). Power walking can burn the same number of calories as running does. Many people want the health benefits and physical exertion that running achieves, but don't want to put such a strain on their bodies. Power walking fits this exact specification.

The benefits of power walking (*see pp12–15*) have led to its becoming a mainstream and extremely popular sport in many countries. It is the most natural form of exercise, it requires very little equipment, and yet it offers so many benefits.

WHY POWER WALK?

Researchers in the field of sports and fitness have described walking as "the activity closest to perfect exercise." It seems far too simple to claim that a basic skill that most of us do without a second thought can be so significant, but as you begin to learn more about your body and the benefits of walking, you will realize that it is true; the action of walking may be simple, but the results for your health and daily living are far-reaching.

Our society is becoming more and more sedentary and overweight. We sit in our cars instead of walking, many of us spend hours seated at a desk at work, and thanks to computers, we can now do a lot of our shopping without leaving home. Not surprisingly, more and more people complain of posture-related aches and pains, and life really is no fun if every day is a battle to find our energy and sparkle. Yet we are missing one vital point. Exercise in any shape or form is an essential part of our lives, not an optional extra that we may or may not choose to do.

Making the commitment

Exercise is often seen as something undertaken to get rid of a beer belly, or to fit back into a smaller dress size, particularly in the summer months. You don't often hear people say that they must do some exercise to clear their mind, or to make them feel happy. Yet in truth, the health of your mind, body, and spirit are all inextricably linked. Imagine yourself as a triangle, supported in each corner. If one support goes, the others are put under tremendous strain to keep you balanced. That challenge is continually happening in our bodies, but walking can help to keep that balance.

Walking alone or with company is the best exercise you can do for strengthened muscles, a healthy heart, a toned body, and a clear, focused mind.

Committing yourself to exercise can be much like dieting; the desire to do it comes and goes in phases. We have all been there. We know we should do it, but we need to be in the right frame of mind. We then get enthusiastic and eager to transform ourselves. We go to the gym or follow a program for weeks or maybe months, feel great, and vow to keep it up. However, for some reason we break the routine, and then suddenly we are back at square one, thinking we must get in shape.

This is a familiar cycle to most people, and just like on-off dieting, it doesn't work. To change this pattern, the first thing you must do is to ask the question, "Why hasn't it worked?" The answer is usually boredom, and not achieving the results and quick fix that you want. A major key to finding a lifelong sport that you can stick to is choosing something that is fun, is motivating, has variety, can be as challenging as you want it to be, achieves physical results, suits your body, and fits easily into your life. Staying active is commonsense body maintenance that will ensure that you can still choose to power walk and enjoy life to the fullest when you are well into your eighties and beyond.

Take a step in the right direction

Just by taking that first step towards power walking, you will be considering your walking posture and helping your back to become stronger and more flexible. Walking is also an aerobic exercise, which means it pumps blood to your muscles to be used as energy. Because walking requires the use of your arms, legs, torso, and many muscle groups, any amount of regular walking will increase your cardiovascular strength. This in turn will increase your ability to do more, without getting tired. By being able to do more, you will also be building muscular endurance, which means you will keep going longer with sustained energy. Imagine flying through all your daily chores and still having the energy to go out and walk a few miles.

THE BENEFITS OF POWER WALKING

Reduces tension, stress, and anxiety, and enhances mental well-being.

Tones and strengthens your muscles.

Improves muscular endurance and flexibility.

Helps manage body weight and reduce body fat.

Boosts your immune system.

Relieves the symptoms of premenstrual syndrome.

Increases bone strength and prevents osteoporosis.

Reduces the risk of cancer.

Improves cardiovascular fitness, which can help reduce the risk of coronary disease and strokes.

Is socially enjoyable.

Detoxes the body and improves skin texture.

Improves sleep patterns.

Eases the pain and stiffness of arthritis.

Reduces the risk of Type 2 diabetes.

Boosts the level of HDL (healthy cholesterol) in the blood and reduces high blood pressure.

Helps you stop smoking and promotes healthy eating.

Improves energy levels and self-esteem.

Relieves and prevents back pain.

Although walking does not exercise all your muscles, it does work hard on the back of your body, in particular your calves, hamstrings, gluteals, upper back muscles, and shoulders. Because your other muscles need to stay flexible and functional, too, I have included in this book some daily stretching exercises and other activities to complement your walking so that you will use your body to its full capacity.

Preventing illness

The impact of weight on your bones and joints as you walk will strengthen them and ultimately protect them against osteoporosis. Although this disease is more common in older people, whose bones become weak and can be vulnerable to fractures, it is never too late or early to build bone density.

Walking will also increase your circulation and speed up your metabolism, which means not only that you will burn more calories but your body will become more efficient at absorbing the nutrients from your food. In turn this will encourage you to drink more water. Insufficient intake of water is the source of many disorders. Drinking more can help to improve your digestion and detoxify and cleanse your system. Among other benefits, this will give you a more efficiently working body and radiant skin.

It may be hard to imagine but it is nevertheless true that walking for 30 minutes a day will bring huge benefits for your immune system. The stronger your immune system is, the more protection against ill health you will consequently have. It is your barrier against absolutely everything that your body has to confront on a day-to-day basis, from the common cold, flu, pollution, and stress to heart disease and cancer, so it is important that you keep it functioning to its optimum level.

The mind-body connection

If you are aware of your body at all, you will know how tired and sluggish you become both physically and mentally if you go through periods of inactivity. Untroubled, natural sleep can often be so elusive. One of the major benefits of power walking that you will notice very quickly is how soundly you sleep. We all need different amounts, but having enough sleep can make you feel calmer, more in control, more tolerant and patient, more enthusiastic about trying new things and challenges, more joyful and content. Restful sleep can be the magic key to the quality of your life.

Stress is another drain on our resources and can lead to all sorts of complaints, from asthma and high blood pressure to depression and anxiety. Walking has been shown to be a positive way of relieving stress and improving self-esteem. It gives you the space to think, solve problems, and gain clarity. Walking in parks or anywhere that feels close to nature will also bring a sense of peace in difficult times.

Premenstrual syndrome may be caused by a physical change, but the effect on mood is something that most women experience. However, walking and exercise can reduce the symptoms and keep your serenity intact.

Life is good

With a healthy body, plenty of sleep, and a clear mind it would be difficult not to have a spring in your step and to feel that life is good. Exercise releases endorphins, often called "happy hormones," which is why you always feel so good after you have been active. Combine that with walking with friends or family and you will have an enriched spirit. Alternatively, if you want to expand your creativity, walk alone and let the energy of nature inspire you.

As your health and fitness levels increase, you will begin to see the excitement in life's challenges. Perhaps these include losing weight, or maybe you will decide to take part in a marathon. The possibilities are different for everyone, but what is the same is that we all need the necessary vitality to be excited by them and to visualize our dreams coming true. I have been able to witness and share enriching experiences with many women and men who originally decided to start power walking just to get fit. Believe me, there is nothing quite as exciting as witnessing flowers bloom.

GETTING STARTED

You don't need to invest in special clothes or equipment to power walk effectively, but good shoes are essential and will ensure that you walk to the best of your ability. This is especially important when you consider that each time the foot strikes the ground, it bears two-and-a-quarter times the body's weight, and that it is estimated that a relatively active person will take 8,000–10,000 steps each day, and walk 83,000 miles in a lifetime.

(The foot is) "a masterpiece of engineering and a work of art." LEONARDO DA VINCI

THE RIGHT SHOES FOR YOU

Our feet are one of the most complex parts of our bodies. Each foot is made up of 26 bones, 32 joints, hundreds of nerve endings, and four layers of muscle that fit between the sole and the top of the foot. In addition, feet come in all shapes and sizes. If we want our feet to perform well, we need to make sure that they have the right footwear to do the job.

How you walk

Most feet fall into one of three walking styles: those that pronate, those that supinate, and those that are neutral. It is important that you know which category you fit into when you buy shoes, since some have insoles built in to correct excessive pronation or supination. To determine what kind of foot you have, try the following wet foot test.

Footprint analysis

Dip your foot in water, shake off most of the excess, and then walk across a large sheet of posterboard, or a dark-tiled floor if you have one.

If you leave a footprint that forms a flat, solid band, with little or no distinction where the arch should be, then you are a pronator. A low arch, or flat feet, can exacerbate this. This is the most common bearing, and while a certain amount of pronation, where the foot rolls inward and the arches flatten, is normal, with excessive pronation (also known as overpronation) there is a pronounced inward roll of the foot as it lands. This can twist the foot, shin, knee, and hip, and can cause stress throughout the body. Other symptoms of excessive pronation are rough skin forming on the inside edge of the foot (the medial) and on the heel.

TREAD WEAR

The soles of an existing pair of your shoes will also reveal your walking gait. Place the heels together so that you can see them at eye level. If the heels are worn on the inside and the shoes lean in, you pronate. If the heels are worn on the outside and the shoes lean out, you supinate. If they are not excessively worn on either side, your walking gait is neutral.

Pronation (left foot)   tread worn on inside   **Neutral** (left foot)   tread worn evenly   **Supination** (left foot)   tread worn outside

If you leave a footprint that shows just the toes, ball of your foot, and heel, then you are a supinator. Supination (also called underpronation) is where the feet do not have enough inward motion, and roll to the outside edge of the foot after landing. As a result, hard skin may form on the outside edge of the foot.

If your footprint is somewhere in between the two, then your feet are neutral (pronation neutral). Here, the foot neither excessively pronates nor supinates, and the center of the heel strikes the ground. The soles of your shoes will also reveal a great deal about the way you walk—study the diagrams opposite to learn more about tread wear.

Causes and cures

There are many causes of excessive pronation and supination, including corns, bunions, and other foot complaints, knee problems, or being overweight. Walking at even a few degrees out from the neutral gait can cause your body to overcompensate and take it out of alignment. To correct excessive pronation, look for a shoe that will support the inside edge of your foot, and has extra stability in the heel. If you are a supinator, ideally you should have a shoe that has good heel stability and extra cushioning under the ball of the foot. If you have a neutral gait, you can wear any good-quality shoe.

It is also possible to self-treat minor pronation and, to a lesser degree, supination by using ready-made corrective insoles, or orthotics. These are designed to support your foot in the necessary places to correct your gait and prevent injury. However, if in doubt, do not attempt to diagnose the problem yourself, but seek advice from a properly qualified chiropodist or podiatrist and get a professional biomechanical assessment of your feet. A foot specialist can also arrange for custom-made orthotics to be created for you.

KEY POINTS TO LOOK FOR

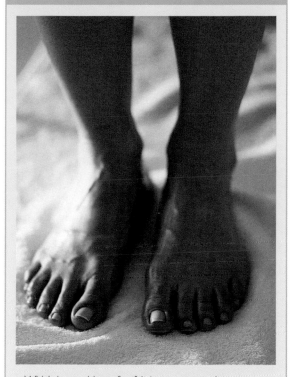

• Which is your bigger foot? It is common to have one foot larger than the other. Buy shoes that fit the bigger foot, and make adjustments to the fit of the smaller foot with insoles.

• Which is your longest toe? Usually, this is the big toe, but sometimes the second toe is the longest. There should be a two-finger width between the end of your longest toe and the end of the shoe (see p20).

• Are your feet wide or narrow? Most shoes come in one width, and while the fit can be adjusted slightly by the way you lace your shoes (see pp22–23), if you have very wide or narrow feet you will need to buy shoes that are sold in different width sizes.

• Do you have a slim heel? This is a common feature in women, and may be combined with a wide fitting across the broadest part of the foot. Lacing your shoe to accommodate a narrow heel may help (see p23).

• Do you have large toe joints or bunions? If you do, you may want to see a podiatrist for expert advice on shoe fit.

Shoes for walking

Many people ask the question, "Can I wear a running shoe for power walking?" Well, you wouldn't expect to perform well if you played tennis in soccer shoes, and the same applies to walking and running shoes. A shoe suitable for power walking must be flexible; at push-off, a power walker's forefoot flexes at nearly twice the angle of a runner's. The shoe needs to be pliable enough to follow the roll of the foot as you lead the heel-to-toe action. A walker lands on the heel, so good supportive cushioning in the heel is essential. The height of the heel on a walking shoe also needs to be on the low side. Many running shoes have quite a high heel, which, when you power walk, can force you to overwork the shin muscles and cause injury.

It is important to find shoes that suit your feet. If you are unable to find a specific walking shoe, a cross trainer or a multi-terrain trail shoe is your next best choice. Aside from the key points (see opposite), a good starting place is to ensure the shoes are flexible, waterproof, and have good grip on the soles.

Shopping for shoes

Choose a specialty athletic shoe store that has a good reputation and trained staff. The staff should be able to assess your feet and direct you toward a selection of shoes that are right for you. The best stores have a treadmill so that you can try the shoes in action; some may even allow you to take a quick "test walk" outside.

Buy shoes in the afternoon. Feet swell slightly throughout the day and when you walk vigorously, so always try on shoes when your feet are at their largest. Take with you a list of your foot details (*see p19*) so that you don't forget any important points about fit. Also make a note of any injuries, past and present. They may have a bearing on which shoe you choose. Study the page opposite and note the key features you should be looking for in your walking shoes. Take your walking socks with you. You should always match your walking socks to your shoes so that they work together. Also take along your orthotics if you wear them. Finally, remember that shoes come in all price ranges, but expensive does not necessarily mean the best for you.

ORTHOTICS

These corrective insoles are designed to change the motion of the foot, in particular to relieve excessive pronation, and to stop further deterioration of the foot for those with flat feet or bunions. Preformed orthotics are available in retail stores, while custom orthotics are made after a biomechanical assessment of your foot by a qualified podiatrist or chiropodist. They are designed specifically for your feet, and may include features such as heel lifts.

preformed orthotics

custom orthotics

WHAT TO LOOK FOR

A shoe suitable for power walking must be light and flexible so that it can mimic the range of movement from the foot. Make sure that the toe box is roomy and rounded so that your toes can move freely; unless you have very slender feet, avoid tapered toe boxes. You will need to have at least a two-finger width between your longest toe and the end of the shoe to allow sufficient space for the push-off movement.

Low-cut heel
Due to the acute angle of the ankle every time you push off, a low heel profile will help prevent pressing against the Achilles tendon and any risk of injuring this very fragile part of the foot.

Lightweight and waterproof
A good walking shoe should be as light as possible, and preferably waterproof, so made from a Gore-Tex material.

Flexibility
Any shoe suitable for walking must be flexible while protective, allowing the foot to have a full range of movement from heel to toe.

Toe box
This area needs to be roomy, deep, and preferably rounded so that your toes have plenty of room to lie flat and protected while at the point of "push-off."

Stability
Whether you pronate or supinate, look for a heel that will provide stability and help to correct the condition.

Arch support
In any good walking shoe, there should be good arch support and insole.

Cushioning
Supportive cushioning is essential, especially in the heel and under the ball of the foot.

When you are trying on a pair of shoes, your feet should feel well supported and protected inside the shoes, comfortable and without any pressure on any part of your feet, held well in the heels, and supported under the arches. It is worth noting that walking shoes, as with most sports shoes, tend to be small for their size, and you will probably need to try on shoes that are anything between one and two sizes larger than you normally wear.

Pay particular attention to the toe box. Some toe boxes can be quite tapered, and unless you have very slender feet, your toes can bunch up slightly. This may feel fine in the store, but as soon as you start to walk any distance, your toes will start to rub against the shoe, causing blisters and bruising. Make sure, too, that there is a two-finger width between your longest toe and the end of your shoe.

You should not have to "wear in" shoes. If they pinch or rub in the slightest way, leave them on the shelf. You want to walk out of the shop ready to go a million miles.

Caring for your shoes

Now that you have the perfect shoes, help them to last. If you get your shoes wet, remove the insoles and dry them separately. Stuff the shoes with

LACING TECHNIQUES
The way you lace your shoes can further improve the fit of your shoes. This is especially useful if, for example, you have a wide foot but a narrow heel.

Always loosen your laces before you slip into the shoes to prevent stress on the eyelets and wear on the heels of the shoes. Tighten your laces from the bottom eyelets, closest to your toes, to the top of the shoe, pulling the laces tight at each set of eyelets before going on to the next set.

The standard crisscross lacing suits most people, and allows you to tighten the laces more evenly than bar lacing. Most shoes have double eyelets at the top. Use them both for a firm fit for a slim foot, or leave the top set unlaced if you have a high instep or a broad foot.

Lacing for a wide foot
To give you extra width across the foot, thread the laces through the bottom two loops or holes as usual. Skip the next two loops by threading the laces up the side of the shoe. In the middle of the shoe, start to lace crisscross again to the top of the shoe.

Lacing for a narrow foot
Lace the first two sets of eyelets as normal. Keeping the laces on the side of their last eyelet, thread to the next hole. Cross the laces over and thread them back through the bar that has been created on each side, pulling in tight. Resume threading crisscross as normal to the top of the shoe.

newspaper to absorb the moisture, and dry them slowly away from direct heat. Remove the paper after a few hours once it has soaked up as much moisture as possible. Don't try to hurry the drying process by putting wet shoes on or near a heat source, such as a radiator, since this will make the materials in the shoe crack and weaken. Do not put your shoes into the washing machine to clean them. Again, this will speed the breakdown of materials in the shoe. Wipe off any dirt with a damp cloth and leave them to air. If your shoes are very muddy, lightly scrub off the mud under lukewarm running water. Then dry them as before.

Don't store your shoes in a plastic bag or box. Leave them out to air between wearings. If possible, buy two pairs of shoes so that you can rotate their use.

Replace your shoes every 500–690 miles (800–1,100km); write the date of purchase inside the shoe so you don't forget. After this amount of wear, they may still look good on the outside, but they will have deteriorated on the inside to the point where they no longer support your foot properly. My shoes usually let me know when they need changing. A really comfortable pair of shoes will suddenly start to give me blisters, or pain in my ankles as the support slackens.

Lacing for a wide or deep arch
Start to lace as normal with the first two sets of eyelets. Skip the next two eyelets in the middle of the shoe, threading the laces up the side of the shoe. Then continue lacing as normal to the top of the shoe.

Lacing for a narrow or slipping heel
Lace your shoe as normal to the second-last set of eyelets. Make a bar on each side as in lacing for a narrow foot. Loop each lace across and through the bar and pull tight. Tie as normal.

FOR HIKING ONLY

I have seen people end up in a lot of pain when they try to power walk in hiking boots. The very features that make hiking boots ideal for carrying you great distances over rugged terrain—the rigid sole, and a firmly supported ankle—will cause major problems to your feet when power walking. Always wear the right shoes.

WHAT TO WEAR

Comfort and practicality are the key qualities you should look for when choosing clothes for power walking. The goal is to enjoy walking and to be totally unaware of what you are wearing—that's when you know your clothes are really working for you. If you are walking in extremely hot or cold weather, turn to pp114–115 to find out more about what to wear in such conditions.

Legs and layers

After shoes, the next most important consideration is what to wear on your bottom half. Ideally, opt for leggings or shorts that are made from a synthetic, or synthetic mix, stretch fabric that breathes and wicks away moisture from your body to the outside of the fabric, where it evaporates. Make sure that they are not too tight around the waist, and check for minimal flat seams. Walkers move with a scissorlike action, so any garments that have thick inside seams, such as jogging pants or jeans, will cause chafing on the insides of the thighs and a great deal of discomfort.

A mistake that many people make when they start power walking is to wear too many clothes on their top halves. Your temperature can rise and fall quite dramatically throughout a walk, so the trick is to wear thin layers. Start with a tank top or T-shirt, then add a lightweight fleece or jacket (*see box, right*). If your second layer has long sleeves, you can tie it around your waist when you are not wearing it. Some manufacturers make jackets that fold into themselves to form a fanny pack, complete with straps and a buckle to fix around your waist, when they are not being worn.

When it comes to choosing fabrics, again, select those made from synthetic materials, that are designed to draw moisture away from the skin, keeping you dry and comfortable. Cotton feels great to put on, but if you tend to sweat and become very hot, it will cling to you and become wet and cold.

Always make sure you have a layer to put on at the end of your walk. If at all possible, wear light or high-visibility colors and garments with reflective strips so that if you are walking at dusk or in the dark, you can be seen easily. (*For more information on walking and safety, see pp116–117.*)

Headwear is another important item of clothing. A baseball cap will keep the sun out of your eyes when it is hot, and retain heat when it is cold. Again, opt for a quick-drying man-made fiber over cotton.

OUT IN THE RAIN OR WIND

• When it is wet, you need a lightweight jacket in a synthetic fabric, such as Gore-Tex, that is water-resistant and allows your body to breathe inside the jacket. This is not the same as waterproof, which will rapidly turn your jacket into a sauna.

• Make sure that the jacket cuffs can be drawn tight to keep water out, and that the back is long enough to cover your rear end and keep it dry. The neck of the jacket should be high enough to keep out drips, and a peaked hood will stop the rain from falling on your face.

• You may also want to wear gloves in a lightweight synthetic fiber, depending on the severity of the rain and the time of year (*see also pp114–115*).

• If you are walking in strong winds, you need a jacket that has a drawstring bottom to keep the wind out. Again, the best fabric for a windproof jacket is a synthetic one, which will be both tough and light.

HIGH-PERFORMANCE WEAR

The science of fitness clothing has come a long way, and while the beauty of walking is that you do not have to have specific clothing, being prepared and selective about what you wear, so that you stay comfortable and dry in all weathers, can determine how much you enjoy your walk.

Using a water bottle holder will allow you to carry up to 25 ounces (750ml), leaving you completely free to focus on your arm movements.

The ideal fanny pack should be able to hold all the items you may need, but be compact enough not to interfere with your walking technique.

Tank or T-shirt
The aim is to stay cool in the heat and warm when it's cold. A high-wicking top that will not absorb sweat makes an excellent base garment which you can then add layers over as necessary.

Gloves
Necessary for the cooler months, choose gloves with touchscreen-compatible fingertips. This will enable you to look at any GPS device without having to remove them.

Head protection
An ear warmer, or preferably a hat, retains heat in winter. A baseball cap is ideal for protection from the sun and keeping rain off your face in wet weather.

Long-sleeved layer
A light, long-sleeved, breathable garment that is also water repellent can provide a layer of warmth when needed. Ensure that the sleeves are loose enough to swing your arms, and if possible has underarm or side zippers that can be opened, allowing air to circulate when required.

High-visibility reflective clothing
For you own safety, be seen at all times, especially at night or in poor weather conditions.

Leggings or shorts
These should have good stretch and fit comfortably with no raised inside seams that can rub.

Sunscreen
Wear a high SPF 30 or above, and preferably waterproof.

A good foundation

All women, regardless of their bust size, should wear a sports bra—it is an essential piece of equipment. It is important to find not only a bra that suits you and feels comfortable, but also one that gives you proper support. The breasts are made of delicate tissue, not muscle. Vigorous movement may stretch or tear the tissue, and once it has been damaged, the tissue cannot repair itself, so a supportive bra is vital.

Make sure that your bra fits you correctly. It is estimated that 70 percent of women are wearing the wrong size of bra, so if you are in doubt, get measured professionally. It is worth bearing in mind that regular exercise will almost definitely change your body shape over a period of time, and your bra size may change, too.

Some sports bras come with a guide as to the type of exercise for which they are most suitable—that is gentle, moderate, or vigorous. I class power walking as moderate to vigorous exercise, depending on your goal. Bras made from synthetic, or a mixture of natural and synthetic, fibers are best, since they have moisture-wicking properties and allow the skin to breathe. Some bras include a silver fiber, which is said to neutralize bacteria in the area. Others are designed to house a heart-rate monitor, a useful feature if you want to wear one.

Buy two sports bras so that having one in the wash does not stop you from walking. Replace a sports bra within 6–12 months, especially if you are walking 3–4 times a week. Over time, it will lose its elasticity and start to feel loose, which is a clear sign that it needs replacing.

SPORTS BRAS

A well-fitting sports bra should feel snug, but not so tight that it affects your breathing. Look for broad, nonelastic straps that won't cut into your shoulders. Padded straps will give extra comfort. Make sure that the chest band of the bra fits firmly around the rib cage so that it doesn't move when you are walking or reaching up.

Light support Compression bras can be worn as outerwear and have cups fitted inside. These flatten the breasts against the body, keeping breast motion to a minimum, and are most suitable for women with smaller breasts. Compression bras often have reflective strips on them so you can be seen in the dark. The "Y-back" panel on the back gives good support for all sizes.

Firm support Sports bras with molded cups that encapsulate each breast give firmer support, and are ideal for women with fuller breasts. Avoid sports bras that hook together at the front, since these tend to allow more breast motion. Look for pull-on types, or ones that hook at the back. The "Y-back" panel again gives good support, and the open design allows a greater area of skin to breathe freely.

Socks

The subject of sports socks is one that never fails to draw debate among power walkers. Some people swear by thin socks, but I personally find they don't give my feet enough protection, and I would always advocate thick socks with extra padding (*see box, below*). Whichever type of sock you choose, stick to synthetic fibers that will wick away moisture and dry quickly; cotton or wool socks can cause blisters when they get wet. Make sure that your socks are a good fit, not too tight and restricting, and reach high enough to cover your Achilles tendon. Replace your socks as soon as you can see that they are wearing thin on the heels or elsewhere. Never wear your shoes without socks. You will soon be complaining of blisters, friction burns, and athlete's foot—not too mention smelly shoes.

LOW-CUT ANKLE SOCKS

These may look elegant, but very low-cut socks are not recommended for power walking. As you stride, your Achilles tendons continually hit the backs of the shoes, and without high ankle socks, you risk getting blisters.

WHICH SOCK TO CHOOSE?

There are so many styles of sports socks to choose from nowadays that I can only recommend that you try a selection until you find the right one for you. You may need to spend a little extra for good walking socks, but they are worth the investment. Nothing beats wearing a great pair of socks in the right-fitting shoes. Always choose synthetic fibers over natural ones; they are better at drawing moisture away from your skin.

Thick sock with extra cushioning

Thin sock

Very fine double-layer sock

Thick socks with extra padding These are my favorite type of socks. They feel soft and luxurious, and have extra padded areas at strategic points on the foot, in the ball and heel, and sometimes over the arch of the foot, too. Make sure you wear them when buying shoes, since thick socks can create a fit difference of up to half a size.

Thin socks Look for minimal or no seams, and make sure they are made from a synthetic fiber. Thin socks made from cotton quickly get wet and lose their softness. Some people find that thin socks cause friction and don't give enough protection to the foot. However, many people do like them, so go with what works for you.

Double-layer socks These are made with two layers of fabric and are designed to prevent blisters. The theory is that as you move, the two layers rub against each other rather than against your foot. I feel that they are more successful for runners than for walkers.

BASIC EQUIPMENT

One of the benefits of power walking is that you don't need any special equipment. As long as you have on a good pair of shoes, you can open your front door and set off. However, for your own comfort and safety, and certainly if you want to keep accurate track of your progress or take part in walking events, there are a few pieces of basic equipment that you will find helpful.

Pedometers, GPS, and Smartphones

Measuring distances has never been easier. You can now choose from an overwhelming amount of devices that can measure anything and everything, either on a specific device or by apps downloaded onto your smartphone. It is all at your fingertips.

A small pedometer or pedometer bracelet are the most basic and are inexpensive and ideal for beginners. These will track key information such as distance, pace, step count, and time. Plus, many will also have a calorie counter so that you can check on energy used during your walk.

Moving up a notch, there are devices designed to be worn 24 hours a day. These will do all of the above, plus keep track of your steps and calories used each day, record your heart rate, track your sleep patterns, and also play music. A smart watch will give alerts via texts and emails, as well as many other features that can support not only your health and fitness, but also your daily life.

You can also download a variety of apps onto your smartphone. The data from your device can be transferred to your app so that you have an instant walking log that will keep track of your week-in, week-out progress.

Your smartphone can make the perfect training partner. The downside is that in certain areas, they can be unreliable as the GPS signal goes in and out. It is also important to be aware that from a safety perspective, they can be very distracting.

Apps

There are a multitude of apps that you can download to support your training. There are individual apps to measure distance and pace, predict calories used, tell you what to eat, measure your heart rate, monitor your sleeping, or motivate you to the next challenge. Depending on the range of support you are looking for, choose apps that combine different features so that you don't have to juggle multiple apps.

When choosing the app that you need, check to see if it is set only by gender, or if it requires personal information, as well as setting your goals and fitness ambitions.

You can download apps to help with everything from plotting different routes to daily Pilates or kettlebell workouts.

10,000-step daily challenge

The goal of 10,000 steps (approximately 5 miles) was dreamt up many years ago. There appears to be no scientific backing to why this distance is better than any other; however, it has now stuck globally as the magic daily distance to be achieved for good health and fitness. Wearing a device every day that counts steps will not only tell you what you are achieving, but also make you very aware of what you are not doing. The average person will take approximately 2,000 steps to walk a mile and a sedentary person may only average 1,000–3,000 steps a day, so choosing a device that will sensitively increase your daily distance can be a very positive step towards many health benefits.

It is common knowledge that being sedentary for too long can be harmful, so your device can also be set to vibrate each hour, or as often as you wish, as a signal to get up and move around. It can also keep you challenged by setting a daily goal.

With the constant encouragement and motivation some wearers can get quite competitive with themselves in the ambition to reach their goal, even if this means going out of their way to make up extra distance. If you want to compete and compare with friends, you can track progress and earn virtual badges for extra motivation. There are also online communities that you can join.

How to fit it all together

Start by wearing the device every day for one week. Put it on in the morning and wear it until bed time. Some people even decide to sleep with it on to study sleep patterns. By the end of the week you will know your average daily steps, which may really surprise you!

It is important to note that the 10,000 steps taken throughout the day should be in addition to any mileage that you complete on your training plan. However, depending on your level of fitness, you may need to gently build up the distances.

Accuracy, versatility, and price are the key points to consider when choosing a device to support your personal training.

Fanny packs and other accessories

You should always wear a fanny pack when you go out power walking, regardless of the distance you intend to walk. You can keep it loaded with all the essentials that you might need, and use it to carry a few first aid items, keys, money, lip balm, sunglasses, and your phone (*see also pp116–117*).

For comfort, make sure that the pack fits into the small of your back to avoid it bouncing up and down as you walk. Ideally, it should come with a water bottle holder either attached or as a separate unit.

If you really do not like to feel anything around your waist, use a wrist or arm pouch. This is a small zipped purse, just big enough to hold keys and money, that has a Velcro strap to fit it snugly around the arm. You can also find arm pouches to hold your phone or device.

Avoid backpacks—they are bad for your posture, and even the lightweight ones will tend to cut into your shoulders after a few miles. However, if you are trail walking (*see pp112–113*), you may want to invest in a nice-fitting, light backpack with well-padded straps.

START WALKING

Before you begin any new exercise plan it is important to determine your fitness and flexibility so that you begin working out at a level that is right for you. By following the easy step-by-step sequences you will quickly develop the correct walking technique. Team these skills with the ability to plan the best routes, and you will be ready to get walking.

"A journey of a thousand miles begins with a single step." LAO TZU

HOW FIT ARE YOU?

Whether you are just starting out or are already quite active, it is important to determine your level of flexibility and strength before you begin a new form of exercise, to avoid overworking your muscles or training harder than is healthy for you. Assessing your fitness for power walking isn't necessarily that obvious. If you do an aerobics class three times a week, you may have good stamina but weak walking muscles, while if you walk to the bus stop every day, you may have strong legs.

Flexibility and strength

Flexible muscles and tendons are achieved through a regular stretching program and by including stretches when you warm up and cool down (*see pp52–53 and 68–72*). A full range of motion is important for everyday life, and more specifically to achieve and enjoy a good walking technique.

The calf muscles, the Achilles tendon, and the muscles down the shin are all used in power walking. To test how flexible you are in these areas, sit on the floor with your legs out in front of you. Flex your feet so that the toes move toward you. If they move beyond the point of being perpendicular to the floor, then your flexibility is excellent. Exactly perpendicular is good, and anything less than perpendicular means that you need to work on improving flexibility in your leg muscles.

Establishing how strong you are will help you to determine what stage you need to start your training at (*see pp52–53*). Core muscle strength is vital for your posture, and good posture and stability are essential components of the power-walking technique. The test on the page opposite will help you to assess your core stability strength.

Check your fitness

The heart is the most important muscle in the body, beating more than 100,000 times a day. This unique engine moves blood from your lungs, where the blood collects oxygen, to the muscles, where the oxygen is burned as fuel. Like any other muscle, the heart needs to be worked to keep it strong and healthy. Cardiovascular exercise, such as power walking, does this by increasing the body's demand for oxygen and making the heart beat faster. Your age and level of fitness are the biggest variables affecting your heart rate. Not drinking enough water while walking, the food you have eaten, tiredness, or anxiety can all cause fluctuations and influence the rate at which your heart beats.

Heart rate and exertion

When you start exercising, it is important to know your level of aerobic fitness so that you work within safe and controlled levels of exertion. Your resting heart rate is a good guide to your current level of fitness. The stronger your heart is, the more blood it can pump through the body with each beat, which means it needs to beat less at rest, and while exercising, compared to the heart of an unfit person.

LOWER BACK FLEXIBILITY TEST

Lower back and hamstring muscles are important in power walking. To test them, sit on the floor with your legs straight in front of you, ankles flexed, and feet flat against a wall. Reach your hands toward the wall. If your palms reach flat against the wall, your flexibility is excellent. Knuckles to the wall is good, fingertips is average, not reaching at all means stretching is vital.

CORE MUSCLES TEST

This exercise assesses strength in the core muscles. If your back is in neutral, flat to your hand, and does not arch as the leg lowers, this is a good indication that you have strong muscles. The weaker your muscles, the more your back will arch (*see pp54–59*). Return to these exercises every so often to assess your progress. Stop the test if it feels uncomfortable at any point to ensure that you don't strain your back.

1 Lie on your back with a neutral spine and place your hands under the small of your back. Inhale deeply, and slowly lift your right leg, keeping the leg straight and the foot flexed. When you breathe out, use your core muscles to slowly lower your right leg. As your leg reaches 45 degrees, feel with your hand to check if your back is arching. Repeat on the left leg.

2 If your back didn't arch in Step 1, try this more advanced move. Start in the same position and lift both legs. As you exhale, slowly lower them and notice what happens to the small of your back. Only very strong core muscles will allow you to lower your legs without any movement in your back.

To establish your resting heart rate, sit down for at least 10 minutes, then feel your pulse on your wrist (the radial artery). Hold your upturned wrist with your thumb underneath for support, and one or two fingers placed lightly on the inside of your wrist. Count the beats of your pulse for 10 seconds, then multiply this number by 6 to calculate the average beats for 1 minute.

A fit adult has a resting heart rate of 50–60 beats per minute (bpm). The heart of an average adult beats at about 72 bpm at rest, and an unfit person has a resting heart rate of 80–90 bpm. Some people, though, naturally have a higher or lower heart rate.

Heart-rate monitors

The most efficient method for measuring the heart rate is to use a heart-rate monitor (*see opposite*). They are simple to use and very efficient. Most take into account information such as your gender, age, height, and body weight to give you a realistic idea of your training zone (*see box, below*).

Once you know your resting heart rate, you can establish what your optimum training zone should be (*see box, below left*). If you are out of shape, you should work at the lower end of your maximum heart rate (MHR), and if you are very unfit, you may need to drop as low as 55–50 percent of your MHR. To continue improving your fitness, increase the intensity within the range of your training zone. A strap-on heart-rate monitor is the most efficient way of checking your heart rate while moving.

The Borg scale

This is a system of numbers to describe intensity in exercise (*see below*). The Borg scale relies on your own perception of exertion—how fatigued or not you feel while exercising—and is therefore a quick way of assessing how hard you are working. It is particularly useful for those at a higher level of fitness who are in tune with their bodies. However, beginners may not find it quite as accurate, since they may feel they are working at a higher rate than they really are.

When walking at a brisk pace, most people should feel they are working between four and seven on the Borg scale. A person of average fitness would feel that seven is an appropriate level of exertion. If you feel you are working too hard, then slow down. If the workout feels too light, try speeding up.

HEART RATE TRAINING ZONE

To work your heart and lungs in the most efficient way, it is important to exercise between 65 percent and 85 percent of your maximum heart rate (MHR). If you are a man, $220 -$ your age $=$ MHR; and if you are a woman, $226 -$ your age $=$ MHR. For example, if you are a 40-year-old woman, your MHR is 186 beats per minute (bpm).

To find your optimum training zone, work out the upper and lower limit percentages:
65 percent of 186 (0.65×186) is 117 bpm
85 percent of 186 (0.85×186) is 153 bpm
The training zone for a 40-year-old woman, therefore, is between 120 bpm and 158 bpm.

Working out above the upper limit would put unnecessary and unproductive stress on your body. Below the lower limit, you may not be working hard enough and may not see any real benefit from your walking program.

Borg Rate of Perceived Exertion (RPE)

RPE	DESCRIPTION
0	Nothing at all
0.5	Very, very weak
1	Very weak
2	Weak
3	Moderate
4	Somewhat strong—endurance training
5–6	Strong—endurance training
7–9	Very strong—strength training
10	Very, very strong
*	Maximal

Place one or two
fingers lightly on the
pulse point _____

The most common type of heart-rate
monitor consists of a chest strap with
a transmitter that measures the
electrical activity of your heart and
then sends radio signals to a receiver
fixed to your wrist. For a manual check
of your heart rate, feel the pulse point
on your wrist (*above*).

To achieve the best results from your
walk, you do not need to push
yourself at 100 percent capacity.
Your ideal pace will work your heart
between 65 percent and 85 percent
of your maximum heart rate.

SETTING YOUR STRIDE

To make the most of power walking as a fitness program, you need to determine your current walking pace. The aim then is to increase your walking speed over time in order to improve your level of fitness. The length of your stride is the important factor here—once you have established the average length of your stride, you can work out how far and how fast you are walking.

Stride length and frequency

The length of your stride is largely determined by the length of your legs. However, the flexibility of your hamstrings, the muscles at the back of your thighs, and the amount of mobility in your hips will also have an impact. If you do suffer from tight muscles, walking and stretching will undoubtedly help to improve this.

A power walker's stride should feel easy and no wider than your usual length of stride (*see pp42–43*). Beginners often assume that to move faster they need to take larger steps, but actually the opposite is true.

As you develop your technique, you will ultimately shorten your stride to increase your speed. This is borne out by racewalkers, whose

WHAT DOES A PEDOMETER TELL YOU?

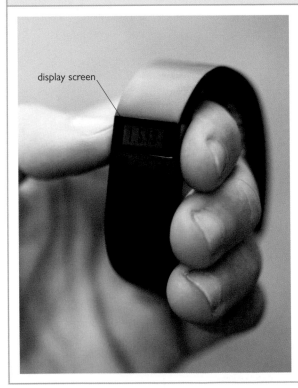

display screen

Many pedometers and pedometer bracelets have a full range of features that are particularly useful for tracking progress on a training walk, monitoring your 10,000 steps, or following a weight-loss program.

Calories This feature will estimate the calories burned based on your weight. This is a great incentive for those wanting to lose weight.

Time Many pedometers have a stopwatch that starts when you take the first step (and can be reset), others also give the time of day.

Speed Some pedometers will calculate your average speed based on how many steps you take per minute.

Alarm This is useful if you are incorporating interval training in your walks (see p136). The alarm can be set to sound as a reminder for you to change your pace. For those in more sedentary jobs, keen to make sure they are active for a few minutes each hour, set a vibration alarm to remind you to get up and move around on a regular basis.

transfer of weight from hip to hip is so quick they can only take very small steps. To begin, try increasing your pace by keeping to a comfortable stride. To quicken your movements, just take more steps per minute. If you feel that you are bouncing or becoming unstable as you walk, the chances are that your stride is too wide. Experiment with a number of stride lengths to find the right pacing for you. You should be able to roll from one foot to another without losing the fluid movement.

Measuring your stride

There are several ways to measure your stride. The first is perhaps the quickest, but is not necessarily the most accurate. Many devices will calculate your stride by your height using one of these simple formulas, depending on your gender.

- Men multiply their height in cm by 0.415
- Ladies multiply their height in cm by 0.413
- For example, a lady 160cm tall: 160cm x 0.413 = 66.08cm (round to 66cm)

Another more reliable way is to measure your stride. You will need a tape measure and a couple of pieces of chalk to mark a line. Make sure you have a space large enough to allow you to get into your natural stride and walking rhythm for about 10–20 strides.

Mark a start line with your chalk and place your heels against this line. Holding the other piece of chalk, take your 10–20 steps forward, getting into a smooth rhythm. After 10–20 strides, stop with your feet together and place the second piece of chalk at your heels. Now measure the distance between your two heel chalk marks. Divide the total distance by the number of steps taken to give you your stride length. For example, if you took 10 steps and the total distance

between the two heel marks is 21ft 4in (650cm), divide this by the number of 10 steps to give your average stride length of 2ft 1½in (65cm).

Over the coming weeks and with regular walking, your stride is likely to alter, so repeat this process again several times to calculate an average stride length. Eventually, your technique and speed will develop naturally and you will be able to work out your walking speed just from experience.

Steps per minute

To estimate the distance you travel without using a pedometer (*see opposite*), you will need to measure your stride. Count the number of steps one foot takes in 1 minute, and then double this figure to get your total number of steps per minute. Now multiply this by your stride length measurement to determine how far you have travelled in 1 minute. The chart below will give you an idea of your current walking pace.

Walking pace	Women	Men
	Minutes per 1 mile (1.6km)	
Easy	17–19 plus	16–18 plus
Moderate	13–16	12–15
Fast	12	11

Depending on your goal, it will also determine the pace you walk. Even though you may set your stride, no walker is restricted to using one walking pace. Interval training, for example, will use all three walking paces and is an excellent way of accelerating your health and fitness. For successful weight loss, the emphasis will be on regular walking a minimum of four times a week rather than pace. However, for endurance or marathon training, it will be important to pump your heart, and therefore make steps per minute the focus.

PLANNING YOUR ROUTE

Great pleasure can be found in spontaneously choosing to go for a walk, but it can also be frustrating. It can be difficult to judge the distance of some walks, which means sometimes a walk can be over too soon, or that you can travel farther than you had intended. The key to an enjoyable and successful walk is to first establish your walking ability, and then map out a range of routes that match your level of fitness. This list will grow over time as your ability improves.

Whatever your fitness level in other activities, if you are new to power walking, you need to discover your walking ability before you plan any routes. The best way to do this is to walk 1 mile (1.6km), and record how long it took you and how you felt when you finished. If you are concerned that this sounds like a long way, bear in mind that people walk an average of approximately 3 miles (4.8km) in the course of a weekly shopping trip.

Measure your ability

The ideal place to test your speed and ability over a controlled distance is on a running or athletic track. These can usually be found in schools or parks, and you may need to ask permission to use one. As a general rule, the inside lane of a standard track has a distance of 440 yards (402m), but they do vary, so always check the length. To walk 1 mile (1.6km), you will need to walk around the inside track four times. As you move outward from the inside lane, each track increases in length by about 7½ yards (7m). A track is useful when measuring your ability because there is no traffic to disturb your concentration; there are facilities such as restrooms and water close by, and it is a safe place to stop if you feel uncomfortable at any time. If there isn't a track near you, the other option is to measure the distance of 1 mile (1.6km) by car or by bike on a road, for you to walk afterward. Try to make it a circular route so that you are never far

from home, just in case you become tired or need to stop.

Walk at your fastest pace, but without straining yourself, and time how long this set distance takes you (remember to warm up and cool down, *see pp68–72*). It may take 15 minutes, it may take 30 minutes or more, or perhaps you will need to stop before the end. When you have finished, assess your progress. For example, could you have kept on walking? Did your legs ache? Was it a struggle, and were you out of breath? The answers to these questions will help you to decide your next move. If you are able to walk 1 mile (1.6km) easily, you are ready to begin one of the programs (*see pp142–187*). When you start your program, listen to your body, and if the regimen feels too easy or too hard, try another one at a different level. Revisit this test after a few weeks to monitor your progress.

If you struggled to complete the course, you will probably want to walk at your own pace and distance for a few weeks to become accustomed to the exercise. For example, try just one lap of the track, or find the ¼- and ½- mile (0.4km and 0.8km) points on your route, see if you can reach one or both of them, and then build up from there.

Moving on

Now that you have established your walking ability, and the distance of your start walk, you need to research two or three routes. Some walks will be more successful than others, and it will take a while to build up a list of your favorite routes. Be realistic—if a route takes too much organization, or if you are unsure of the area, then you simply won't walk it. It is important that you enjoy the surroundings. Accessibility, variety, and enjoyment should be your guides when planning walks.

Urban walking

One of the benefits of city walking is that there are usually plenty of level sidewalks, which allow for a constant stride pattern. There may also be city parks, schools with sports fields, or even rivers or canals to add variety to your walking routes. Do some research about your town to see if you can create a route that will pass some historic features. Check out local maps to see if there is a lake you could walk around, a state forest with hiking trails, or a picturesque view that you could enjoy. Use power walking to explore your local surroundings and offer you new experiences.

The negative side of city walking is concerns about safety. For more information on how to walk safely, see pp116–117.

Mall walking is another popular option. The benefit of walking in malls is that they provide a safe, climate-controlled environment, complete with facilities. The network of main thoroughfares and side aisles will give you plenty of scope to vary your routes, and to make them as long or as short as you want. Try to avoid busy times of the day so that you don't intimidate shoppers and can allow yourself plenty of room to walk. Many shopping centers unlock their doors especially for mall-walkers before the stores open each morning.

The great outdoors

If you live in a rural area, your routes may include anything from farmland and wooded areas to forests, hills, and coastline. There is nothing quite like walking in the country, with the calming sights and sounds of the natural world all around you. You may find, too, that spotting birds and other wildlife along the way can pleasantly distract you from the effort that you are putting into your workout.

Walks in the country will give you a slightly different, possibly harder, workout if the route involves you walking on dirt tracks or up hills as opposed to flat, even surfaces. Recreational paths are fine to use in your route, but you may need to watch your footing and keep your eyes (and ears) open for fast-moving cyclists. Both hills and uneven paths will make your muscles work harder over the same distance; bear this in mind if your walk feels tougher than you expected.

There may be less traffic and pollution out of town, but if you walk on a road with no sidewalk or shoulder, you still need to watch and listen for cars and be ready to step off the road if necessary.

STEPPING IN THE RIGHT DIRECTION

Vary the length of your routes. Even advanced walkers will want shorter routes for when they have less time.

Include surroundings that will match different moods, from the tranquillity of a park to the bustle of a busy street.

Decide whether you want your walk to start from your front door, or whether you are willing to take public transportation out to a new area and walk from there.

If you're walking at night, make sure the area is safe, with good sidewalks and streetlights. Even during the day, avoid known trouble spots.

Some routes may have heavy traffic and pollution at certain times of the day. Avoid these times if possible.

Establish if there are restrooms and stores to buy water if needed on the route, and their exact location.

If your walk goes through a public park, check the opening times.

POSTURE AND BREATHING

The use of modern technology in the workplace has led many of us to become more sedentary than ever before, our bodies hunched over desks, reinforcing the very muscles that create poor posture. The best antidote to this is an activity such as walking, in which good posture and breathing are an essential part of the exercise.

Functional posture

Our core muscles in the back and abdomen (*see pp52–53*) are responsible for holding our bodies upright. However, without constant and proper use, these muscles become lazy and stop working efficiently. Then, when we do try to stand tall and have good posture, it can feel awkward and uncomfortable because the muscles are being asked to do something they are not used to. Standing tall, try drawing your navel into your spine using your natural corset and notice how your spine automatically realigns. If you do this regularly, you will not only begin to improve your posture, but you will also strengthen and flatten your abdominal muscles, stand taller, and have a more defined shape.

The head-neck-back relationship is key to good posture. The body follows the head, so if your head juts forward, your spine will follow suit, straining the muscles in the neck, shoulders, and

POSTURE CHECK

Notice how your muscles feel as you bring your body into neutral position.

Incorrect posture The head is thrust forward, chin jutting out, straining the muscles in the neck and shoulders. The shoulders are slouched and the chest is collapsed. The abdominals are pushed out, arching the spine and throwing the pelvis back.

Correct posture Make sure your weight is evenly distributed, the toes spread to form a stable base. Imagine a straight line from the heel through the back of the knee (not locked). The hips are tilted forward and the bottom is tucked under. The chest is raised, the shoulders down and relaxed, the neck softly extended. The chin is parallel to the floor and the crown points to the ceiling. The spine is in neutral, which means it is allowed to retain its natural curves.

eyes looking down

Collapsed chest affects oxygen flow

abdominals are pushed out

look straight ahead

chest is raised and open

hip tilted forward

back of knee directly above heel

feet slightly apart

upper back. People who sit a lot, especially in front of a computer, have a tendency to protrude the head and neck forward.

Often, when people start power walking they complain of lower back pain and blame it on the exercise when in fact it is caused by poor posture. It is important to correct posture as early as possible because as we age, bad posture can contribute to all sorts of health problems, from chronic headaches to arthritis.

Breathing

The act of breathing is so natural and automatic that most of us don't give it a second thought. Yet few of us breathe correctly. In general, people use shallow, or chest, breathing and do not use the full capacity of their lungs. Poor posture, too, can restrict the rib cage and prevent the lungs from expanding properly.

> **TIP** A good friend gave me this simple tip to correct posture. Attach an elastic band around something you look at often during the day, such as your telephone at work. Each time you see it, spend 30 seconds squeezing your shoulder blades together. Persevere with this and it will become second nature, strengthening your upper back muscles and in turn helping improve your posture.

Breathing deeply using the diaphragm when you are walking will help you to get the most out of your sessions (*see pp76–77 for more on diaphragmatic breathing*). But first you need to get in touch with your breath and experience the energy it brings. Try the breathing exercise below, and as you breathe, mentally send oxygen into the body. Feel the sensation of directing air in and out while the spine lengthens. Practice this until you are able to recreate this feeling when you are out walking.

BREATH AWARENESS

Lie on your back. Lengthen your neck by bringing the chin slightly towards your chest. Your eyes are open and looking straight ahead. Feel your belly button pulling toward the spine. Place one hand on your abdominals just below your navel and the other on your rib cage. Breathe in slowly and rhythmically and be aware of the corset muscles working. Do not allow the abdomen to pop out. Breathe out and feel the sensation of your rib cage moving. Widen the shoulders and feel the shoulder blades moving slightly toward each other. Experience the whole of your upper body broadening rather than moving upward.

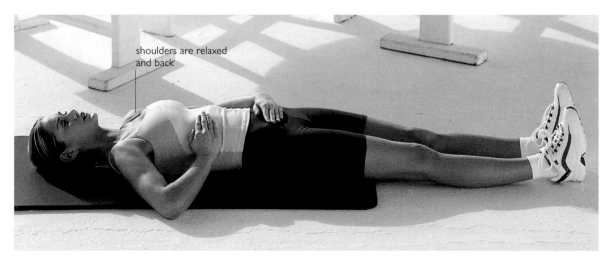

shoulders are relaxed and back

POWER LEGS AND FEET

A few minor adjustments to the way you walk will allow you to easily make the transition from regular walker to power walker. The action of power walking requires that the pelvis and hip area move freely so that the legs can stride out, followed by a pronounced rolling heel-to-toe motion as you move forward. Work on achieving a good heel strike and a dynamic push-off.

1 Stand tall, shoulders relaxed and back, your midsection pulled in, pelvis tipped forward. Hold your arms loosely by your sides. Now extend your left leg, taking care not to lock or over-extend the knee. Flex the left foot so that the toes point upward.

2 Take a normal stride length and place your heel squarely on the ground with a really good upward lift on the ankle; this will give you a full range of movement as you roll the left foot through to the midstance position in Step 3. Your right, back foot is firmly planted on the ground.

3 Move forward onto the left foot so that your weight is evenly balanced between the heel of the left foot and the ball of the right foot. Look straight ahead, chin parallel to the ground, and remember to keep your shoulders relaxed.

WALKING A LINE

As you take each step, imagine that you are walking down an imaginary line. Your feet should be placed almost directly in front of each other, rather than a wide stance. This saves time and energy as you walk.

4 Transfer your weight onto the left foot, keep the leg straight, and keep the weight on your left heel for as long as possible before rolling the length of the foot. Begin to rise onto the ball of the right foot ready for the push-off—the most important part of the power walk. The power and thrust comes from pushing off from the toes. It's a challenging move, so begin by exaggerating the push, and feel your leg extending fully from your toes. You may lean forward slightly at this point.

5 Begin to cross through to the front with the right, back leg and keep the foot close to the ground. Neatly step the foot through; avoid big movements, which waste energy and time.

6 Extend the right leg immediately while raising the foot slightly in preparation to strike with the heel, as in Step 1. As you practice, allow your arms to swing naturally in opposition to your feet (*see also Power Arms pp44–45*).

POWER ARMS

This strong arm movement contributes to a compact and streamlined body, allowing you to move rhythmically and efficiently. Often, people feel self-conscious when they start using power arms, but you will find they are your source of energy and are essential to achieve speed. If you are troubled by poor circulation, good technique will help your hands to stay warm by keeping the blood pumping through them.

1 Stand tall, with your arms relaxed by your sides in the beginner's position. As you start to walk, your arms will naturally swing in opposition to your feet. Experiment with the intensity of your swing as you begin to power walk. Throughout, make sure that the swinging motion starts at your shoulder.

2 This is the neutral position. Your elbows are bent at a 90-degree angle and sit lightly on your waist. Your hands should be relaxed and gently cupped. From the beginner's position in Step 1, progress to walking with your arms in this position. Your elbows shouldn't move as you walk; the movement is from the shoulders.

make sure arm
doesn't cross
the body

tuck elbows
into sides

hand no lower
than waist height

Both hands should
be lightly cupped.

3 When you are ready, start using full power arms. To practice, swing your left arm forward until your hand reaches no higher than shoulder height. Simultaneously bring your right arm back, your hand just brushing your waist. Both arms should be square to the body and elbows bent at 90 degrees. Move with purpose. In this optimum position, the front, leading arm should feel as though you are punching the air, while the back arm moves with force, as though you were elbowing someone behind you.

WEIGHTS AND WALKING

I advise against walking wearing wrist or hand weights because they put a strain on the elbow joints and can create risk by raising the blood pressure. For an occasional arm workout, try carrying two half-filled small bottles of water. Keep sipping from both of them so that by the end of your walk the bottles are empty.

PUTTING IT ALL TOGETHER

Combining power legs and feet with power arms may feel a little awkward at first as you try to keep track of what your feet are doing while making sure, for example, that you don't bring your arms up too high. The only way around this is to start walking and keep practicing.

1 Begin with a strong, upright posture, your torso lifting from your hips and midsection, eyes looking straight ahead. Check that your shoulders are relaxed and your chest is open. Stand with arms in the neutral position, with elbows bent at a 90-degree angle and hands lightly cupped.

2 Stride forward with the left leg, the left ankle well flexed, and ensure that the right, back foot is firmly planted. Start to move the right arm forward and the left arm backward, in opposition to the feet. As the left heel strikes the ground, begin to transfer your weight from the right foot onto the left foot.

3 At the midstance position, your weight is evenly distributed between the ball of the right foot and the heel of the left foot. Continue to move the arms toward their optimum positions. Make sure that you are looking ahead.

4 Transfer the weight fully onto your left foot as the right foot lifts onto the ball, the toes ready to give you a good push-off that will generate your speed. Feel a strong extension in your right leg, your body leaning forward slightly. At the same time, work your arms to propel you forward, the right arm punching forward and the left arm "elbowing" backward. Watch that your front hand doesn't go higher than shoulder height, and that the back hand doesn't dip below waist height.

5 Lift your right foot and keep it close to the ground as you begin to transfer it to the front. Start to move your right arm backward and your left arm forward, again in opposition to the leading foot.

6 Extend the right foot forward, the toes raised, heel ready to strike; remember to keep your feet pointing forward as if walking an imaginary line. Swing the arms through the neutral position and into the next cycle.

COMMON MISTAKES

Some of the problems that walkers develop may arise from poor posture. If you suspect that this is true for you, reread the information on posture on pp40–41. If you feel that you are slipping into any of the faults shown below, try checking how you walk in front of a mirror at home and make some adjustments, or ask a friend to watch you while out walking and give you pointers to improve your technique.

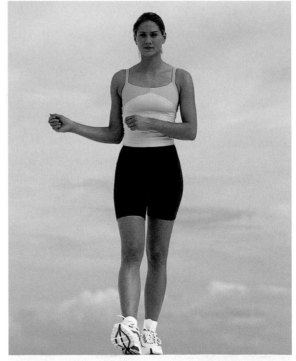

Wide and open

This is a common fault, where the arms hang loosely out to the sides, and the feet are wide. Men in particular have a tendency to walk like this. If the lateral muscles are overdeveloped, it is awkward to hold the arms close to the sides. People walking with a wide gait tend to point their toes out to the sides, and consequently the feet roll out to the side. Actively think about how you are using your feet.

Juggling arms

Here, the arms are bent at the correct angle, but as they move, the arm going backward swings out to the side, while the leading arm crosses the body. Keep your arms square and at an equal width apart at all times. The arms should not cross the centerline of your body. Keep your elbows tucked in to your waist.

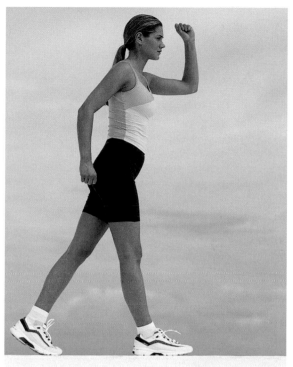

Leading arm too high

As the leading arm goes too high, it also becomes too wide and open, and you may find that your feet follow suit. Work on condensing the action of both arms and restricting the thrust of the leading arm.

Leaning forward

This fault can stem from poor posture, but I suspect that many people lean forward in the hope that they will travel faster. Bending forward forces your eyes to look to the ground, which is bad for your posture and can cause injury. Look straight ahead of you and your posture will naturally realign itself. Leaning forward is often accompanied by another fault: taking too-large steps. The assumption here is that overstriding will move you faster, but it has the opposite effect—the smaller the steps, the faster you will move. To remedy this, keep your arm movements small and your feet will follow.

QUICK GUIDE TO GOOD TECHNIQUE

• Maintain good posture, using your midsection.

• Ensure a strong upward lift on the ankle of the leading foot as it moves to the heel strike.

• Take normal-length strides—don't overstride.

• The heel of the leading foot is planted squarely in front of the back foot.

• Push off well—this is your power point.

• Work your arms from the shoulders, and keep the elbows at right angles at all times.

• Keep your movements compact and streamlined.

STRETCH AND STRENGTHEN

Combining power walking with regular stretching and strengthening exercises will enhance your walking ability and make you more body-aware. As you discover how your body works, you will come to appreciate the importance of maintaining core stability. The following moves will start you on the road to stamina, poise, balance, and a strong and agile body. As soon as you are ready, expand your repertoire of exercises, drawing on Pilates, yoga, exercise ball routines, and strength training.

"Truly a flexible back makes for a long life."
CHINESE PROVERB

WHY STRETCH AND STRENGTHEN?

Our muscular system works as a whole to enable us to perform controlled movements efficiently and without stress. For example, when you power walk, you are using all the muscles that run from the gastrocnemius muscle in the calf to the sternocleidomastoid muscle in the neck. Yet from the half-hearted way that many people stretch before and after exercise, it seems few of us appreciate the interdependent relationship between muscle groups, and it's not often that you see someone doing neck stretches before going for a walk.

The muscles responsible for movement are known as skeletal, or voluntary, muscles, and they can act in two ways: they can contract and shorten, or they can relax and lengthen. Most skeletal muscles work in pairs. The muscles are attached to bones, so when one muscle group contracts, another muscle group lengthens, pulling the bones together or apart and creating movement. Muscle groups are either mobilizing—creating motion—or stabilizing—holding and supporting while other limbs are moving. This is why it is so important to stretch opposite muscle groups, such as calves and shins, and hamstrings and quadriceps.

Flexibility and stretching

Being flexible means that you have good mobility in your muscles and joints. Many factors will have an impact on your flexibility, including your level of activity and whether you work in a sedentary job.

HOW OFTEN?

You should always stretch when you go for a walk (see *Warm-Up and Cool-Down*, p72). If you can, also stretch on days when you are not walking (see *also Walking Programs*, pp140–187). For strength, ideally do all the exercises on pp54–59 two or three times a week. There is also a program of stretching and strengthening you can follow on p73.

Muscles and joints also become less flexible with age. The way to improve your flexibility, and relieve tension, is through stretching exercises. Before and especially after an activity, stretching (*see pp68–71*) is vital to elongate muscles that have contracted through use. Regular stretching, even for just 10 minutes a day, is a good habit to get into, whether or not you have been exercising.

To get the most out of your power walking, you need flexibility in the muscles you use most: your hamstrings, calf muscles, Achilles tendon, and the muscles in your shoulders and upper back, which you use in the strong power walking arm movement.

Core strength

The core muscles in the back and abdomen (*see page opposite*) help us to stand up and function correctly. In particular, the abdominal muscles, which wrap around the torso and connect the rib cage to the pelvic girdle, keep the core of the body stable and maintain posture. When these muscles are contracted, they act like a corset, keeping the back and front of our bodies in alignment. If these muscles are not used regularly, as in a sedentary lifestyle, they become weak, which leads to poor posture and even shoulder and back problems. By investing in keeping good flexibility and strength, we are not only helping ourselves to stay in shape but ensuring a long and active life.

WALKING AND POSTURE MUSCLES

The muscles in bold are all the postural muscles that cross all the weight-bearing joints. All these muscles enable you to stand erect and power walk.

Sternocleidomastoid

Deltoids

Pectorals

Biceps

Serratus anterior

Oblique abdominals

Abdominal corset

Iliacus
Psoas

Adductors

Quadriceps (quads)

Tibialis anterior (shins)

Trapezius

Deltoids

Triceps

Latissimus dorsi

External obliques

Erector spinae

Gluteus maximus (glutes)

Hamstrings

Gastrocnemius and Soleus (calf muscles)

Achilles tendon

DOUBLE LEG STRETCH

This sequence is taken from Pilates. The Double Leg Stretch is a beginner's exercise and is ideal for strengthening the lower abdominal muscles and for challenging your coordination. If you have any problems with your lower back, in Step 2 straighten your legs up to the ceiling instead of holding them at 45 degrees.

1 Lie flat on the mat with your knees bent and arms out to the side, palms facing downward. Draw both knees up and into your chest, bringing one hand to each leg, with toes pointed. Now use your abdominals to lift your head and shoulders off the floor. Do not allow your arms to help you lift your upper body. Arms are soft, with elbows out to the sides. Keep your neck long and support it by bringing your chin toward your chest, but maintain some space between them.

keep legs straight

Do not let your head fall back

torso is kept still

2 Inhale, and reach your arms back behind your ears and stretch your legs out at a 45-degree angle from the floor. Squeeze your buttocks and inner thighs together to support your back. As you stretch your body, imagine that you are being pulled in two directions, with only your abdominals holding you firmly in position on the mat.

3 Exhale and draw your knees toward your chest. Move your arms in a wide circular movement out to each side. Sink your belly deeper into the floor as though you were trying to squeeze all the air from your lungs. Repeat the sequence 5–10 times. End the exercise by returning to Step 1 and exhaling deeply.

SINGLE STRAIGHT LEG STRETCH

This exercise is also taken from Pilates and can be done on its own or following the Double Leg Stretch. It is a more advanced move that strengthens your core muscles and elongates and strengthens the muscles at the backs of the legs. Start slowly, but with practice the action should be quick, smooth, and rhythmic.

1 Lie flat on the mat with your knees bent and arms out to the side, palms facing downward. Draw both knees up and into your chest, bringing one hand to each leg, with toes pointed. Now use your abdominals to lift your head and shoulders off the floor. Keep your neck long and support it by bringing your chin toward your chest, but maintain some space between them.

2 Inhale, hold your left ankle with both hands, and extend your leg to the ceiling. Stretch out your right leg and hold it at about 45 degrees from the floor. If you cannot reach your ankle, move your hands up your leg (but do not hold behind the knee), and raise the lower leg to a comfortable height. Contract your abdominals and press them into the floor to support the weight of the lower leg—do not use your shoulders for support. Exhale as you switch legs in a scissor action and hold the ankle of the right leg. Repeat the sequence 5–10 times and end by bringing both legs back to Step 1.

toes are pointed

keep head and shoulders lifted

knees are straight but not locked

ROLLING THE BALL

Working with an exercise ball is a great way to improve your core strength and stability. If you have not used an exercise ball before, take the following exercises slowly and make sure you feel confident in each position before moving on to the next step. Work on a soft surface and be prepared to roll around. If you have a back problem, seek expert advice before attempting this exercise.

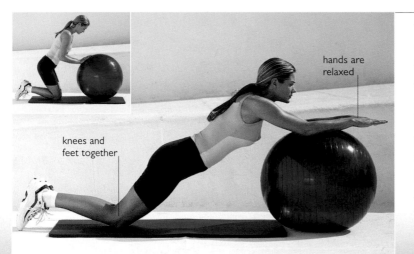

knees and
feet together

hands are
relaxed

1 Kneel facing the ball, hands flat on the ball, arms bent at the elbow. Roll the ball forward a short distance until your forearms are resting on top of the ball (you may have to build up to this). Contract your abdominals to support your torso as you balance between your knees and the ball. There should be a straight line from your shoulders to your hips. Hold for 5 seconds, then roll back. Do 2 sets of 5–10 rolls, resting 1 minute between sets.

2 Once you are proficient in Step 1, move on to this more advanced position. With forearms still resting on top of the ball and a neutral back, rise up onto your toes and aim to have your body as straight as a plank. Hold for 5 seconds, return to Step 1, and rest briefly. Complete 2 sets of 5–10 sequences, with a 1-minute rest between sets.

keep neck long

pull in
abdominals

THE BRIDGE

This exercise also improves your core strength and stability. It works your core muscles and also your glutes and hamstring muscles. Even if at first you don't reach the position in step 2, you will still get a good workout by attempting it. For an advanced workout, lift each leg as described in Step 2. If you have a back problem, seek expert advice before attempting this exercise.

1 Lie on your back, with your arms relaxed by your sides, palms facing downward. Widen your shoulder blades (*see breathing exercise, p41*). Rest your legs together on the exercise ball so that your heels and calves are comfortably positioned.

2 Using your core muscles, raise your hips and pelvis so that your body forms a straight line from your shoulders to the tips of your toes. Pull in your buttock muscles and feel your abdominals pressing toward your spine. Keep breathing and hold the position for 15–30 seconds, then return to the start position. Complete 2 sets of 5–10 raises, with a rest of 1 minute between sets. When you are ready, from the raised position, lift one leg off the ball, hold for 5 seconds, then raise the other leg. Watch that your pelvis stays square and does not sink toward the floor.

MODIFIED BALL POSITION

If you feel you need more stability to begin with, place the ball against a wall so that it is kept stationary as you do the exercise.

BALL CRUNCH

The secret of balancing on the ball is to calm the mind, focus on the precise stabilizing point, and make small correcting adjustments. This exercise opens your chest, stretches your spine, and really works your abdominals. If you have a neck or back problem, please seek expert advice before attempting this exercise.

open your chest

use thighs for support

1 Sit on the ball and walk your feet forward until you are lying back on the ball with your knees bent at 90 degrees. Feet are flat on the floor, hip-width apart. Let your head lie back over the ball. Open your arms wide and let them fall toward the floor. Draw in your core muscles to support the pelvis.

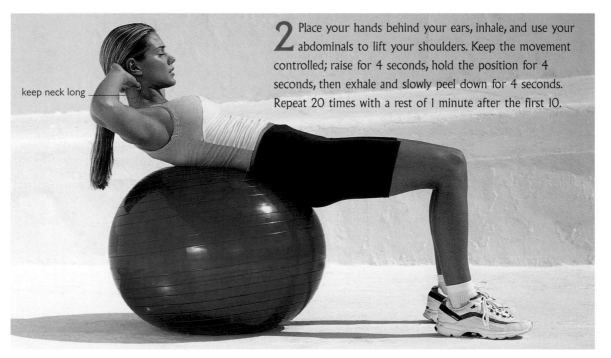

keep neck long

2 Place your hands behind your ears, inhale, and use your abdominals to lift your shoulders. Keep the movement controlled; raise for 4 seconds, hold the position for 4 seconds, then exhale and slowly peel down for 4 seconds. Repeat 20 times with a rest of 1 minute after the first 10.

SUPERMAN

This exercise is challenging because it requires great control, strength, and balance. Start slowly and play around with each position. Remember that you will still be working your core muscles while you are wobbling and practicing the positions. If you have a back problem, please seek expert advice before attempting this exercise.

1 Lie face down over the ball with your back in neutral. Hands are flat on the floor with arms shoulder-width apart. Feet should be hip-width apart, but at first have them at a width that feels right for you. Find your exact balancing point on the ball— when you find it, you will feel steady and secure.

2 Hold your balancing point. Use the power in your core muscles to raise your shoulders and upper body away from the ball. Stretch your arms out to the sides to help you to balance. Feel your chest opening and expanding. Steady your breath and use it to assist your balance in every step of this sequence.

3 Raise your left arm straight in front of you, in line with your body. Straighten your right leg out behind you. Use your core strength to hold yourself still. Look straight ahead, hold for 5 seconds, then switch arms and legs. Repeat on each side 5–10 times.

4 This position is the ultimate in using the pivotal point of balance and takes practice to get right. Raise both your arms and legs. Give the "thumbs up" sign to activate your shoulder blades for balance. Hold the position for as long as you can, then rest.

UPPER-BODY STRETCHES

The upper body, shoulders, arms, chest, and particularly your neck can hold a great deal of tension, which can cause stiffness. Stretching restores good mobility and releases a great deal of stress. These upper-body stretches are subtle but effective. They should feel pleasurable, so if they are painful in any way, you are pushing too hard. Be aware of having good posture before beginning each stretch.

Neck Stretch

Stand tall with your feet slightly apart and knees soft. Move your arms behind your back, with your right hand lightly clasping your left wrist. Keep shoulders straight and gently ease the left arm toward your right arm. You should feel the stretch at the front of the left shoulder. Hold for 10 seconds and repeat for the other arm.

Neck Stretch: Position 2

Tilt your head to the right as you ease the left arm toward the right. You should feel a stretch all the way down the left side of your torso. Hold for 10 seconds, then repeat the entire sequence on the other side.

Triceps Stretch

Stand tall with knees soft and legs hip-width apart. Raise your left arm above your head and bend it so that your hand is pointing down your spine. Place your right hand on your left elbow and gently ease your left elbow backward to get a good stretch in the back of your arm. Hold the stretch for 10 seconds and then repeat for the other arm.

Shoulder Stretch

Stand tall with knees soft, and reach up with both arms. Feel a stretch lifting from the pelvis all the way up to your fingertips. Keep your right arm raised and bend it so that your hand is pointing down your spine, palm facing in. Drop your left arm, bend the elbow, and interlink the fingers of both hands. Check that your back is in neutral and not arched. Feel the stretch through both shoulders while you hold for approximately 20 seconds, then repeat with opposite arms.

BEGINNER'S ALTERNATIVE

If you are unable to reach far enough to interlink your fingers, hold a belt or small towel to bridge the gap; gradually work at bringing your hands together.

Upper-Back Stretch

This stretch releases tension in the upper back, shoulders, and neck. Kneel on the floor with knees approximately hip-width apart. Lean forward to place your hands in front of your knees, palms facing downward. Walk your hands forward and away from you until your arms are outstretched. Feel the stretch through your spine from your pelvis and deep in your shoulders. Hold for 15 seconds and then return to a sitting position.

ALTERNATIVE

Poor flexibility and tightness in your shoulders and upper back can prevent you from doing the full stretch. If this is the case, fold your arms on top of each other and rest your head on your arms. Open your shoulder blades and feel a gentle stretch in your upper back.

LOWER-BODY STRETCHES

The muscles and joints in the legs, pelvis, and lower back are going to work hard while power walking, so they need particular attention. It is important to build strength in vulnerable areas, such as knees and ankles, to reduce the risk of injury. You will receive greater benefit from your stretches if you focus on the muscles you are stretching. Little but often is the best policy with these stretches.

Hip Flexor Stretch 1

Stand tall with your feet hip-width apart, then take a step back with your left leg. Place your hands on your right leg for support just above the knee. Lunge slowly forward onto your right leg, keeping the knee at 90 degrees and above the heel. Keep the hips square and ease them forward by tightening your buttocks, feeling the stretch in the front of the hip. Hold for 10 seconds and repeat on the other side.

Hip Flexor Stretch 2

Take a normal-length stride forward with your right foot. Keeping the knees bent, rise onto the balls of both feet, as though you were wearing high heels. Keep your hips square and ease them forward by tightening the buttocks, feeling the stretch on the front of the hip. Hold for 10 seconds and then repeat on the other side.

Achilles Tendon Stretch

Stand tall with your feet hip-width apart, then take a step back with your left leg. Lean forward on the right leg into a deep lunge as though you were going into the original Hip Flexor Stretch. Then rise up onto the ball of your left foot to create a good stretch for the Achilles tendon. Hold this for 10 seconds and repeat on the other leg. This stretch works well when completed following Hip Flexor Stretch 1.

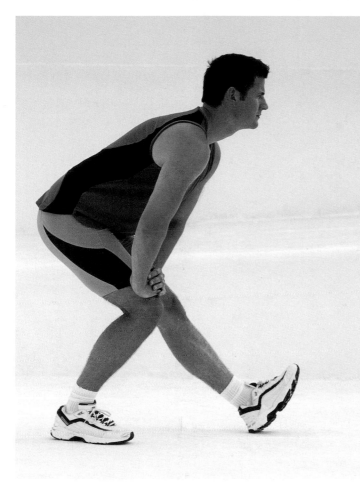

Hamstring and Calf Stretch

Stand tall, with your feet together. Step your left leg forward a normal stride-length. Stand with your right foot flat on the floor, toes pointing ahead and left foot flexed. Bend your right knee and place both your hands at the top of your right thigh to support your weight. Lean forward slightly onto your right foot and sit back into the position. Feel the stretch in your hamstring and calf. To intensify the stretch, sit farther back. Hold for 10 seconds and then repeat on the other side.

ALTERNATIVE
Begin the stretch as above, but keep the left foot flat on the floor. This is a gentler stretch for the hamstring and creates a stretch down the shin.

Ankle Stretch

This stretch is taken from yoga, and it is ideal for power walkers because it strengthens the ankles, knees, and hips and increases flexibility in these areas. Sit up straight, with the soles of your feet together. Grasp both ankles and bring your heels as close to your body as you can. Allow your knees to fall toward the floor—this will get easier with practice. Stay like this for 10 seconds, or longer if you find it comfortable to do so and enjoy the position.

Be sure your feet are touching from toes to the heels.

FULL-BODY STRETCHES

The Side Rolls rotate the spine and stretch your obliques (the waist muscles). To advance the Side Rolls, grip a tennis ball between your knees. This will keep your pelvis straight and stretch your obliques more intensely. The Back Stretch gives the spine a powerful stretch and opens the chest.

keep neck long

shoulders are flat
on the floor

abdominals
pulled in

Side Rolls

Lie flat on the mat with your knees bent at a 90-degree angle, knees close together. Stretch your arms out to the sides, palms facing downward. Inhale deeply, and as you exhale, slowly turn your head to the right. At the same time, slowly and in a controlled movement roll both legs to the left. Hold the stretch for about 15 seconds, return to the start position, and then repeat on the other side.

Back Stretch

Lie face down and place your hands directly under your shoulders, with elbows bent and arms close to your sides. Push up from your hands, but keep your elbows bent at around 90 degrees. Hold for 10 seconds, feeling the stretch all the way down your back. Avoid this exercise if you have any sensitivity or problems in your back.

keep shoulders relaxed

ADVANCED STRETCH

From the lying position, push up with your hands as before. Continue to raise your chest and shoulders, lifting from your hips and midsection, until your arms are straight but your elbows are not locked. Your shoulders should be relaxed, shoulder blades dropped down. Hold for 10 seconds, then return to the start position.

BEFORE AND AFTER WALKING

Warming up and cooling down are essential to prevent aches and injuries to muscles during and after exercise. A short routine will aid flexibility and increase the blood flow into working muscles. Once the muscles are soft and warm, stretching will lengthen them and can help train them to become more pliable. Far from being unrewarding or unnecessary, these exercises are a vital part of your walking program.

Warming up

Warming up prepares the body for exercise. As you gently exert yourself, your temperature rises and your blood begins to move more rapidly toward the muscles that are being used, which increases their flexibility. Tight muscles are underused muscles and are prone to injury.

If you are quite physically fit, begin your warm-up by walking at an easy pace for 5 minutes. If you are planning a long, demanding walk or if you are out of shape, you will need a minimum of 10 minutes. Keeping your eyes focused on the path ahead, start to loosen your shoulders and the upper body as you walk, rolling your shoulders a few times. Swing your arms in circular movements and an exaggerated pendulum motion. Your lower body will become warm from the movement of walking. Focus on your body and become sensitive to how it is feeling at that moment. After 5–10 minutes, find a suitable spot to stop and follow the Warm-up

Sequence (*see p72*). Hold each position for no longer than 10–15 seconds. Breathe deeply and relax into each position as you do it. There should be no pain or pressure, just the sensation of your muscles lengthening. When you have finished, continue walking, increasing your pace gradually over the next 5–10 minutes. If you feel tight during the walk, slow down and stretch again.

Cooling down

The longer and more intense your workout, the longer your cool-down will need to be. It is not a good idea to abruptly stop walking because this can cause dizziness.

Five to ten minutes before the end of your walk, begin cooling down. Slow your pace, and once again roll your shoulders and swing your arms. When you stop, follow the Cool-down Sequence (*see p72*). This time you can make the stretches deeper and more intense, holding the positions for 15–30 seconds. Take deep breaths and, as you exhale, send the energy to the muscle you are stretching and let the breath take away tension. Do not bounce, since this can cause strains. Take care not to overstretch because this can cause a weakness in your joints. It should feel comfortable, not painful. If you know that you have weak areas, work specifically on those places. End your session by relaxing in the corpse pose on p71 (not always possible, but a treat when you can).

MIND AND BODY

Warming up not only prepares your body for movement, it also puts you in the right frame of mind for exercising. After a hard day's work, for example, the last thing you feel like doing is pounding the streets. A few minutes of gentle walking and stretching has a miraculous way of changing your mind. Conversely, cooling down allows you time to calm and center yourself before launching back into life.

THE TREE

This yoga position is a personal favorite. It is good for developing your balance, and like so many yoga postures, it also calms and refreshes the mind. Although it is an unusual choice, I find it is excellent for cooling down and becoming centered. To help you balance at first, place one hand on a wall for support.

drop your shoulders

keep chest open

hips square

1 This exercise should be done in bare feet. Stand tall in a good posture with your feet just slightly apart, your toes spread and your weight evenly balanced between both feet. Transfer your weight onto your left foot and clasp your right ankle. Place the heel of your right foot as high as possible on the inside of your left thigh with your toes pointing down.

2 Focus on an object in front of you, and stretch your arms out to the sides at shoulder height to help your balance. Keep the right knee pointing out to the side and your hips straight. If you feel comfortable, raise your arms in a wide, open gesture toward the ceiling. Keep strong and rooted, yet flexible and relaxed. Hold this position for about 10 seconds and then repeat on the other side.

BACK STRETCH

A supple and flexible back is important for your health and fundamental to any movements that you make. Our backs can become tight, not only from lack of use but also from stress, so spend just a few minutes each day repeating these exercises, which will benefit your power walk and day-to-day health.

keep knees straight, but not locked

2 As you exhale, slowly fold forward from the pelvis and reach out with your hands. Place your hands on the wall so that your spine is parallel to the floor. Feel the stretch through your back.

arms are soft

3 Exhale deeply and allow your body to drop toward the floor. Feel the stretch down your back and the backs of your legs. Hold for a few seconds, then slowly curl up along the length of your spine to return to a standing position.

1 Stand tall with your feet together, a stride length from a wall. Inhale and raise your arms above your head, reach tall, and lengthen your spine.

Calf Stretch

Stand tall and position yourself
facing a wall or doorway. Press the
ball of your left foot against the wall
with your ankle at a steep angle.
Keep hips square, facing front and
directly above the heel. Inhale deeply;
then, as you exhale, ease into the
stretch in your calf. Hold for a few
seconds, then repeat on the other
leg. Alternate legs, stretching for
a total of 5 times on each leg.

Corpse Pose

This yoga pose can remove stress
from the spine, leaving the body
calm and centered. Lie on your
back with your legs slightly apart,
arms away from your body with
palms facing upward, eyes closed.
Allow your body to feel soft
and relaxed. Imagine your breath
reaching areas of tension. Remain
in the pose for up to 10 minutes,
then stretch your arms, roll onto
your side, and slowly come up
into a sitting position.

WARM UP AND COOL DOWN

These sequences are essential to prepare the muscles and then return them to a resting state. Warm and lengthened muscles work more efficiently. Cooling down leaves your body lengthened and reduces the soreness you sometimes feel after exercise.

Warm-up Sequence

Walk at an easy pace for around 5 minutes and then do each of these stretches in the order shown. Hold each position for 10–15 seconds. Distance walkers and those beginning a fitness program will need to walk for 10 minutes before stretching.

Neck Stretch *p60*

Triceps Stretch *p61*

Back Stretch *p70*

Hip Flexor Stretch *p64*

Achilles Tendon Stretch *p64*

Calf Stretch *p71*

Quad and Ankle Stretch *p127*

Cool-down Sequence

Begin your cool-down by slowing your pace 5–10 minutes before the end of your walk, then do each of these stretches in the order shown for a full cool-down. To ensure a deeper stretch, you need to hold each position for 15–30 seconds.

Hip Flexor Stretch *p64*

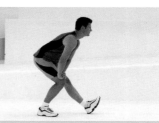
Hamstring and Calf Stretch *p65*

Quad and Ankle Stretch *p127*

The Tree *p69*

Upper-Back Stretch *p63*

Shoulder Stand *p77* (*optional*)

Corpse Pose *p71*

STRETCH AND STRENGTHEN PLAN

Stretching daily will keep you flexible, and strengthening is an essential part of your regimen. The whole program should take around 30 minutes. For a shorter program, use either line one or two and finish with line three, or even create your own plan.

Shoulder Stretch *p62*

Back Stretch *p70*

Lunges *p137*

Calf Stretch *p71*

Quad and Ankle Stretch *p127*

The Bridge *p57*

Ball crunch *p58*

Rolling the Ball *p56*

Ball squats *p131*

The Tree *p69*

Ankle Stretch *p65*

Side Rolls *p66*

Single Straight Leg Stretch *p55*

Upper-Back Stretch *p63*

Corpse Pose *p71*

INNER STRENGTH, OUTER POWER

The more you become aware of your body, the more you may come to appreciate that what you eat and drink, and even the way you breathe, can affect your daily health, energy, and vitality. Examine your attitudes and beliefs and take positive steps to reach your goals.

"Where does the body end and the mind begin?
Where does the mind end and the spirit begin?"

B. K. S. IYENGAR

THE POWER OF BREATH

Breath is life. We can live for weeks without food, days without water, but we can survive only minutes without oxygen. Yet most people are not getting enough of this vital force. They habitually take very shallow breaths through the mouth, and use only the top of the lungs, depriving the body of oxygen. By breathing more fully and deeply we can gain more energy, vitality, and enthusiasm for life. It will not only enhance how we walk, but also contribute to our emotional well-being too.

The mind-body link

The act of breathing has a strong mind-body connection. We know that our state of mind can affect our breathing patterns. When we are frightened or angry, our breath speeds up and becomes irregular. In a totally relaxed state, our breathing becomes slow and rhythmic. In the same way, how we breathe habitually can affect our mood. Shallow breathing through the chest closely resembles the breathing of someone in a state of anxiety, and disrupts the right balance of oxygen and carbon dioxide needed for a relaxed state. Ancient yogis remind us that when the breath is deep and calm, the mind is still, and to achieve this most of us have to work on improving our breathing.

The demands of exercise

It can be quite a struggle, for example, when we are exercising and we find ourselves puffing and panting away. The key is to practice proper breathing before working out, and once on the move, to focus on inhaling and exhaling rhythmically so as not to hyperventilate, which deprives the body of oxygen. The body needs more oxygen when you exercise, and you will find that you naturally increase the number of breaths you take per minute, but you should still maintain a rhythmic cycle of breathing. There is no more exhilarating feeling than when your shoulders are back and relaxed, your chest is open, and your breathing is deep and easy—you will feel that you could walk effortlessly for a hundred miles!

Abdominal breathing

To oxygenate the body fully, we must breathe deeply using the diaphragm (children breathe like this naturally). This is often referred to as diaphragmatic or abdominal breathing.

The diaphragm is a muscle situated between the chest and abdomen. When you breathe in, it moves down to make room in the chest for the lungs to fill with oxygen. As you breathe out, the diaphragm moves up, reducing the chest size, and squeezing air out of the lungs. You are breathing correctly when your abdomen swells forward as you breathe in, and gently falls as you breathe out, and there is little or no movement in the chest area. Remember, breathing out is just as important as breathing in. The more stale air that you can get rid of as you breathe out, the more clean air you can take in.

CALMING THE BREATH

If you are anxious or your breathing becomes erratic for some reason, try this exercise. Sit upright on a chair, your legs uncrossed, feet flat on the ground. Take a slow breath in through your nose for 3 counts and a long breath out through your mouth for 6 counts. Repeat this breathing cycle until you feel more calm.

SHOULDER STAND

This yoga pose is one of the most important for keeping the body in perfect harmony. It also encourages deep abdominal breathing by limiting movement at the top of the lungs. Do not do this pose if you have high blood pressure, breathing difficulties, or back problems.

1 Lie flat on the mat, your knees bent, arms by your sides. For a few moments, breathe in through your nose and out through your mouth, making a soft "ah" sound on each exhale. Inhale and roll your hips off the mat while supporting your back with your hands, your knees at right angles to your body. Exhale.

ALTERNATIVE
As you roll up, use a wall for balance. Take one leg away from the wall and then, when you feel stable, the other.

2 Inhale and take your legs straight up into a vertical position. Try to lift as much of yourself as possible onto your shoulders. Breathe slowly and deeply as you hold the position. Be aware of each breath and how it feels to you. Bring your chin as close as possible to your chest and keep your back straight.

3 To come down, bend your knees toward your head. Straighten your arms in preparation for rolling your body back onto the mat. Slowly peel your body down, vertebra by vertebra, into the start position. Stay there for a few moments, aware of how you feel and what is happening to your breath.

THINK POSITIVE

Although the focus here is on using positive thinking to achieve your fitness goals, you can apply the principles to any area of your life, including your work, your relationships, your self-image, and your health. The power of the mind to affect physical health has been much talked about, but is there any proof? Well, psychologists have discovered that people who feel positive about aging live an average of 7½ years longer than those who see only its downside.

Clearly, the power of thought can have a big influence on our lives, for better or worse. We all hold a constant inner dialogue, or self-talk, that can switch from positive to negative and back again. We often choose the negative path, telling ourselves that we are going to fail or that things won't go right. This prevents us from looking forward to events with happy anticipation, and we may even end up bringing about the very thing we fear.

That negative inner voice can not only prevent us from having the optimism to try to achieve our full potential, but it can also affect our health. Research in Canada carried out over 30 years shows that patients who expect to do well after an operation recover more quickly than those with a pessimistic attitude.

Taking control

So how can we change our attitudes to use the beneficial power of the mind? The first step is to become aware of the nature of our own self-talk.

DROPPING NEGATIVE LABELS

Reframe your thoughts by changing how you view yourself and how you describe yourself to other people. For example, saying "I'm stupid" will in time make this part of your identity. Instead, think in terms of behavior, which can be changed. You may sometimes do stupid things, but no one is infallibly wise. Forgive yourself for your mistake and think of the successes that can be balanced against it.

Psychologists believe that an average person experiences between 20,000 and 60,000 thoughts per day. None of these thoughts are neutral: they are either positive or negative, and they will reinforce themselves day after day.

If you are one of the people who always sees a glass as half empty rather than half full, you need to make a change to positive self-talk to describe your life as you would like it to be. A good way to begin reprogramming your self-talk is to repeat positive affirmations (*see pp80-81*). Make them realistic, so that you can say them with sincerity, and phrase them in the present tense. For example, instead of saying, "In six months, I will be ready to tackle a marathon," say, "Each day I am healthier and stronger."

You will greatly increase your chances of success if you not only believe 100 percent that you will achieve your goal, but also have a goal that is realistic and achievable, one that is challenging for you but not impossible.

However, it is important to remember that positive thinking will not magic away all bad things, and it won't do your training for you! Nevertheless, it will help you stick with the program and deliver the results you want.

A positive outlook affects your body language, making your posture, your walk, and your gestures strong and powerful rather than tentative.

MEETING THE CHALLENGE

We all have dreams and ambitions of how we would like our lives to be, yet all too often, when we consider turning them into reality, we become overwhelmed. We will often try to convince ourselves of many good reasons why we should not try: we don't have the time, or we are not in good enough shape, or we don't have sufficient money, for example. What we probably mean is that we are afraid of failing, or just apprehensive about stepping into the unknown.

Knowing how to take the first step toward meeting a challenge is what separates those who successfully achieve their goals from those who don't. With the right attitude and simple techniques, any one of us can make the changes we want, and work toward achieving our dreams; it just takes practice and courage. As the actress Ruth Gordon once said, "Courage is very important. Like a muscle, it is strengthened by use."

Setting goals

Many of us set out with great enthusiasm to exercise and get in shape, lose weight, or achieve other forms of self-improvement. At first we are dedicated and motivated, but then our resolve begins to slip. We might miss a workout, and once we have done that, it is all too easy to skip another. Perhaps we might succumb to a large slice of chocolate cake and then think that we have gone back to square one, so now we might as well have a second slice.

Setting end goals and expecting to reach them in one giant, unspecified leap is setting yourself up to fail. Instead, if taking part in a marathon is your ultimate goal, the first step is to ask yourself how physically fit you want to be, what kind of finishing time you wish to clock in, and whether you need to make changes to your diet. Be clear on what your objective is and be passionate about wanting to achieve it.

> ### POWERFUL AFFIRMATIONS
>
> The affirmations you use are a personal choice, but here are some favorites of mine that you may like to adopt for your own use:
> - "I am the best I can be in every way."
> - "All of my wishes are now coming true for the good of all."
> - "I am surrounded by love and friendship."
> - "I can do anything I put my mind to."

The second step is to look at where you are now. What is your level of fitness, strength, and stamina? Do you exercise? What will you have to do to prepare for this challenge? How much time can you put aside to work toward your end goal?

The third step is to break down your journey from the present to the end goal into small, manageable pieces. Set easy-to-attain goals so that you will have the constant encouragement of having met them successfully.

Writing down your goals will help you to visualize them more clearly and to see them as a contract you have made with yourself. Each contract fulfilled will boost your motivation to move on to the next. Write them using the present tense, since phrasing them as "I will…" allows your subconscious mind to see them as events that will always be in the future rather than goals to be met now.

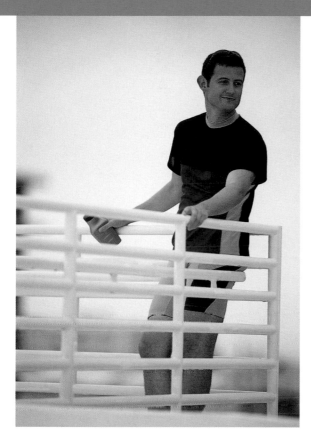

These principles hold good for every area of your life, whether it be weight loss, house renovation, or the advancement of your career; only the details of the goals need to change. For fitness through power walking, create a training plan that includes weekly or even daily mini-goals that perhaps mark your speed or distances. Imagine you are creating a path of stepping stones; each of your stones is a mini-goal achieved, taking you one stride closer to your ultimate success.

The power of your mind

We already know the importance of positive thinking if we are to succeed, but our minds are fickle; it is not always easy to keep our thoughts on the matter in hand. One powerful tool to help you here is affirmations (*see also p78*). Using this technique will help you to stay positive, focused, and believing in your own abilities.

Don't let your dreams remain unfulfilled. Take simple steps to meet your goals, look down from the peak of success, and congratulate yourself on the journey that now lies behind you.

Always affirm the positive things that you desire, not negative outcomes that you are wanting to prevent, and keep them personal and in the present tense. Have only two or three affirmations at any time, giving each one time to work on the subconscious. It is the constant repetition of affirmations that produces the results, and there is no better time to do them than when you are out walking. Let them fall in tune with your step, and repeat them over and over again, rather like a mantra (*see p82*).

Visualizations

Like affirmations, practicing visualizations is about conditioning your mind by repetition, but this time using images and sensations rather than words. You may find it easier in the beginning to close your eyes so that you are not distracted by the reality around you. The more you practice, the clearer the images will become and the more your subconscious mind will accept them as the truth, banishing any underlying negativity that may be holding you back.

For example, if you are planning to take part in a marathon, imagine yourself reaching the finish line, smiling and strong. Feel the breeze on your face as you walk and hear the crowds cheering you on. Think about the clothes you are wearing and how they feel against your skin, and imagine the surge of joy that courses through you when you receive your medal at the end. Try to create a full-color picture in your mind, including every little detail exactly as you want the experience to be. This is visualization, and the more times you return to this powerful image, the more likely it is to become reality.

MINDFUL WALKING

Meditation is sometimes referred to as an act of mindfulness—that is, the mind is focused on a single point or activity in the present moment. Most people assume that to meditate you must sit cross-legged on the floor with your eyes closed, but it is just as possible, if not easier, to meditate while walking. In fact, walking with awareness in the present moment is a wonderful way to spend time walking alone and can bring great emotional and physical benefits.

The benefits of any type of meditation are well documented and include bringing an inner balance, reducing stress levels, and improving sleep. Being mindful and focusing on your breath while power walking is a powerful combination, blending those advantages with fresh air and the acquisition of physical fitness.

Awareness of your movement

Pick a route that is familiar to you, preferably flat, with an asphalt surface, and with little or no traffic, so that walking is easy and distraction is kept to a minimum. Begin your meditation walk by doing a few slow stretches. As you begin to walk, just be aware of the day, the sky, your surroundings, the weather, your energy. Tell your mind that for the next 30 minutes or so, you give yourself permission to be totally in the moment.

Pay close attention to your feet and be aware not only of the contact with the ground as your heel strikes it and your balance shifts to the ball of your foot before lifting off again, but also the the contact between your toes and the feel of your sock fabric.

Next, shift your awareness to your ankles, calves, knees, and thighs. Notice the way your hips lift and fall as you move, and the swaying of your spine. Feel your belly as the center of your being and note the intake and output of breath from your chest. Relax your shoulders and enjoy the rhythm and power in your arms and legs as they move together.

With a balanced head position (*see pp40–41*), you will feel the muscles in your neck relaxe and elongate. Relax your jaw and let your eyes be gently focused ahead. If something distracts you, simply notice it and return your attention to your walking.

Repeating a mantra

Another way to keep your mind in the present moment is to repeat a mantra. This is a word, or group of words, used to keep the mind peaceful and settled. Choose a mantra that feels comfortable and relevant to you, and that will allow your feet to fall into a rhythmic step with each word. While I was going through my cancer treatment, I discovered many, but my favorite is "I am fit—I am healthy."

Repeat your mantra for at least 15 minutes, letting the words fill your head and your feet. There will be times when you will lose your concentration and busy thoughts of the day's tasks and activities will intrude, but quietly put them to one side and reconnect with your mantra.

As you reach the end of your walk, end your meditation and reconnect with your surroundings. Once you have mastered mindulness while power walking, you will find that you have a restored sense of balance and a mind that is perfectly still.

Looking ahead of you as you walk, take pleasure in the rhythm and swing of your arms and legs as they move smoothly in relation to each other.

WATER

The human body can survive for weeks or even months without food, but without water we would die within days. On average, our bodies are made up of between 65 and 70 percent water, though that rises even higher in very physically active people, such as athletes, who have a higher proportion of muscle tissue and less fat tissue. Water is our very life source, and the amount we drink is crucial to our health—yet many of us regularly drink too little.

Statistics show that as many as one person in four does not drink enough water and is dehydrated. We lose around 3 quarts (liters) a day through our urine, feces, sweat, and breath, and although we absorb some water through our food, we need to drink 1.5–2 quarts (liters) a day to replenish that loss. Too many of us drink tea, coffee, or caffeinated soda to quench our thirst, but large quantities of these actually have a diuretic effect instead, as well as being bad for our health. One study has shown that six cups of coffee a day causes a 3 percent loss of water from the body.

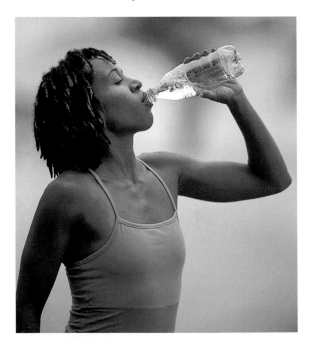

Ensuring that your body is well hydrated will help to keep your skin youthful, your eyes clear, and your digestive system working well. It will also aid in the speedy elimination of toxins from your body and deter cellulite.

Are you drinking enough?

In hot weather, or when we exercise, our bodies dispel heat by means of sweating; during intense activity such as a football game or tennis match, fluid loss can be more than 4.5 quarts (liters) an hour, together with a loss of essential body salts such as sodium, potassium, calcium bicarbonate, and phosphate. When you are power walking, particularly if you are taking part in a marathon, it is important to remember to increase your intake of fluids.

Some experts in sports medicine believe that it is a mistake to use thirst as your guide, and that by the time you actually feel thirsty, you are already dehydrated. Other symptoms of dehydration are irritability and a lack of concentration. Two signs that you are drinking enough water are if you urinate regularly and your urine is a very pale straw color. Make sure you are properly hydrated before you begin walking.

You will need to replace the fluids you have lost by sweating when you have been power walking, particularly when the weather is hot.

Know your water

Drinking water is essential to maintain good health, and it is better to drink water from any source than not at all, but not all waters are of the same quality. The purer the source of the water, the more you will benefit from it.

Filtered water

Activated carbon and ceramic filters reduce the level of impurities in your water, including chlorine, heavy metals such as lead, and sediments, and they will remove the smell and taste of chlorine. Their effectiveness is dependent on the size of the holes in the filter; the smaller they are, the better.

Purified water

The most effective means of purifying water is by an under-sink reverse-osmosis system, which removes about 99.9 percent of contaminants in water, including chlorine, fluoride, nitrates, and lead. The most efficient systems combine activated carbon filtration (*see above*) with the semipermeable reverse-osmosis membrane.

Bottled waters

These come in many guises, and it is useful to learn how to read the labels and become selective. Opt for water in hard plastic bottles or, better still, in glass, since some types of plastics can leach chemicals into the water.

Mineral water This is thought to be the best choice because it is natural and untreated, and must come from an officially registered source. The label will show the mineral content of the water.

Spring water The content of spring water varies from country to country, and in some cases it is a mixture of natural and treated water. Be aware that some bottled waters are very high in sodium and inorganic minerals such as sulfates or potassium, which in this form are not easily assimilated into the body.

> **TIP** When you get tired of plain water, you can always flavor it. I like to start each day with a cup of hot water with a squeeze of lemon or lime added. This is a great wake-up call for the system. A comforting drink on cold days is to pour boiling water over a slice of raw peeled ginger and let it infuse for 5 minutes. For summertime, leave the ginger-infused water to cool, then chill.

Carbonated water Carbon dioxide gas is added to water in order to emulate natural sparkling mineral water. The carbon dioxide inhibits the growth of bacteria, but once consumed, it turns into carbonic acid, which can contribute to acidity problems in the body.

Oxygenated water This is water to which oxygen has been added. The promise is that this will somehow supply the muscles with more oxygen, thereby enhancing performance. However, so far there is little scientific evidence to support this claim.

Bottled tap water In the US, if the label states "from a municipal source" or "from a community water system," you can be sure it is simply tap water.

Tap water

The domestic water supply in most developed countries is subject to more tests and monitoring than bottled water. However, many people are wary of the chlorine used for disinfecting tap water because it can destroy the healthy bacteria in our guts. Pesticides and herbicides used at the source can also leach through into the water supply.

Synthetic estrogens in our water supply, derived from the contraceptive pill, HRT, and plastics, are another concern, since they are thought to be affecting both human and animal fertility.

You can find out more about the quality of your tap water from your local water company.

HEALTHY EATING

Starting to power walk may be the start of reviewing your whole approach to food. As your body grows stronger and more vital, you will want to nourish it with food that gives you the energy you need. The idea of consuming high-calorie, low-nutrient junk food will begin to seem less attractive, as will diets that promise speedy weight loss in exchange for cutting down on the fruit, vegetables, and carbohydrates that your body needs.

It often seems that being healthy is associated with depriving ourselves of the foods we love, but in fact good nutrition is a matter of becoming aware of what we are eating and making choices. Coming to grips with a healthier diet is very simple. Ask yourself two key questions: "Did it once have roots in the soil?" and "What happened to your food before it reached you?"

Foods with roots

Without a doubt, the very best and most nutritious of all our foods are those that started life with roots; they are full of phytochemicals and micronutrients that not only supply our bodies with everything they need, but are also easier to digest and absorb than any other foods. Every time you eat, whether it is a sandwich, pasta, or Sunday brunch, always make sure that at least two thirds of the food on your plate started life with roots in the soil.

If the goal is to maximize the amount of plant-based foods that you eat, then it is also to reduce the foods that do not have roots, such as meat, dairy products, and saturated fats. The latter are normally of animal origin and tend to stay solid at room temperature. Eating too much saturated fat raises cholesterol levels in the blood and can increase the risk of coronary heart disease, strokes, and various cancers.

You should also avoid partially hydrogenated and hydrogenated vegetable oils found in hard and semisoft margarines. These highly processed fats contain synthetic saturated fats known as trans-fatty acids, which have also been linked to heart disease. Many products contain hydrogenated fats, including bread, cakes, doughnuts, cookies, ready-made meals, and even french fries from fast-food outlets.

Nevertheless, our bodies do need some fats to help in the absorption of vitamins and to give us essential fatty acids (EFAs). The polyunsaturated and monounsaturated fats derived from plants, as well as the omega-3 fatty acids from fish oils and flaxseeds or flaxseed oil, aid brain function and cell growth. These fats can then act as a preventative against heart conditions and possibly cancer.

What happened to your food?

When it comes to buying food, what we get is often a lot more than we can see. For example, wheat is sprayed with fertilizers and other chemicals many times, and then, unwashed, is made into our bread. Our humble lettuce looks harmless, but it can be contaminated with a cocktail of artificial chemicals. The ready-prepared foods that are so handy when we come home tired from work are often high in salt, preservatives, and other additives. Wherever possible, buy foods that are organic and prepare them at home. Substitute refined products such as white flour, rice, and pasta with whole-grain versions.

Aim for the best

It is unrealistic to imagine that because you decide to change your diet you will never succumb to another chocolate or fried breakfast. My philosophy is to be selective when you have these treats and make informed choices. If you eat chocolate, eat the best organic chocolate, and if you have a fried breakfast, use the best ingredients with little or no oil. Treat coffee the same way. Use freshly ground organic coffee beans, and savor each sip. This may mean forgoing your regular brew from the coffee machine at work, but if this means you drink less coffee, all the better. Make it a rule to yourself to have the best to be your best.

Eating our seven servings

Experts now suggest that eating a minimum of seven portions of vegetables and fruits a day could lower the risk of cancer by 25 percent and heart disease and stroke by 31 percent, with vegetables seeming to give more protection than fruit. But many of us are unsure of what equals a portion. In fact, a serving is approximately $2^{3}/_{4}$ oz (80g). The following are some useful examples of what constitutes one serving:

- 1 medium apple
- 1 medium banana
- 1 orange
- ¼ cup dried cranberries
- 5–6 baby carrots
- 1 cereal bowl of lettuce
- 1 tomato
- ½ cup broccoli
- ½ bell pepper
- ½ large zucchini

Wherever possible, choose foods that are full of the nutrients that you need—for example, fish for omega-3 essential fatty acids, and nuts and vegetables for protein, calcium, and vitamins.

VITAMINS AND MINERALS

We are often told that if we eat a well-balanced diet with five servings of fruit and vegetables per day, we will get all the vitamins and minerals we need—but medical opinion is divided, with some nutritionists believing that modern-day living requires us to supplement our diet. Certainly, in our busy lives it can sometimes be difficult to fit in those five servings, but we can boost our intake of vitamins and minerals on a daily basis by drinking juices and taking nutritional supplements.

Vitamins and minerals are essential for good health. Although we can manufacture a few vitamins in our bodies, we extract most of the vitamins and all of the minerals we need from our food. Although we require only minuscule amounts, a single deficiency

can be dangerous; most famously, sailors used to succumb to scurvy until it was discovered in the eighteenth century that regularly eating citrus fruits would prevent it.

Vitamins cannot be assimilated into the body without minerals. Together, these two vital substances, along with carbohydrates, proteins, fats, and water, provide you with all the essential nutrients for cell growth, tissue repair, organ function, energy production, and food utilization.

Fruits and vegetables are a rich source of vitamins and minerals, although vegetables do have the edge, with more nutrients. Once again, Jane Sen has a suggestion as to how you can gain maximum benefit, and that is to "shop by color." By reaching the checkout with a basket full of different-colored produce, you will not only have the fun of consuming a wide variety of foods, but will also be giving yourself a huge amount of nutrients.

Natural supplements

Unfortunately, many of the foods grown today have depleted vitamin and mineral content as a result of intensive farming practices, and there is a further loss during transportation and storage. Organic food fresh from the soil is the ideal—and

Blended drinks made of fruit and vegetable juices are packed with vitamins, minerals, and enzymes to boost your energy. They are a delicious way of increasing your water intake, too.

even when our intake of nutrients is sufficient, they can be easily destroyed by factors such as stress, smoking, taking antibiotics, and living in a polluted atmosphere. Opinions vary as to whether taking nutritional supplements is useful or not, but my own view is that they contributed to my recovery from cancer. A high-potency multivitamin and a separate dose of vitamin C would suit most people, but it is advisable to visit a nutritionist for advice or carry out some research into your own requirements first. Buy the best-quality supplements you can afford—the better brands usually have superior ingredients in well-balanced doses compared to cheaper brands—and make sure that the ingredients are from natural sources. Avoid synthetic vitamins,

which can cause toxic reactions and can actually contribute to poor health.

The benefits of juicing

Raw fruits and vegetables that have been juiced retain vitamins and enzymes that are often destroyed in the cooking process. Juicing machines and juicing attachments for food processors are now widely available, and the more expensive models will produce the best results with the tougher and stringier vegetables. Many are hard to clean, so check this aspect before buying or juicing may come to seem like a chore.

There are many books on juicing in which you can find combinations for specific purposes.

WHERE TO FIND SOME OF YOUR MOST IMPORTANT VITAMINS AND MINERALS

Vitamin A	Apricots, cabbage, carrots, egg yolks, cod-liver oil (from an uncontaminated source), mango, melon, spinach, squash, sweet potato, yellow bell peppers, watercress
Vitamin B group	
B1 (thiamine)	Beans, bran, most vegetables, whole grains, yeast
B2 (riboflavin)	Eggs, leafy green vegetables, mushrooms, tomatoes, wheat germ
B3 (niacin)	Cabbage, cauliflower, mushrooms, tomatoes,
B5 (pantothenic acid)	Alfalfa sprouts, avocados, broccoli, cabbage, celery, eggs, lentils, mushrooms, squash, tomatoes
B6	Bananas, broccoli, brussels sprouts, cabbage, cauliflower, lentils, nuts, onions, squash
B12	Eggs
Vitamin C	Citrus fruits, broccoli, cabbage, cauliflower, kiwi fruit, melon, papaya, peas, peppers, sprouted seeds, strawberries, tomatoes
Vitamin D	Egg yolk
Vitamin E	Beans, broccoli, raw leafy green vegetables, peas, pine nuts, sunflower and sesame seeds, unrefined corn oil, wheat germ, whole-grain cereals
Folic acid	Avocados, broccoli, cashews, cauliflower, hazelnuts, spinach, walnuts, wheat germ
Calcium	Almonds, brewer's yeast, cabbage, dried beans, green vegetables, nuts, sunflower seeds
Iron	Dates, dried beans, egg yolks, miso, nuts, oats, pumpkin and sesame seeds
Selenium	Brazil nuts, broccoli, cabbage, lentils, mushrooms, wheat germ, zucchini
Zinc	Almonds, Brazil nuts, brewer's yeast, egg yolks, oats, pumpkin seeds, rye, whole wheat

FOODS FOR FITNESS

Your diet won't turn you into an athlete, but it will help your body to perform at its best. Exercise burns up energy in our bodies, and to achieve results, it is important to make sure that you have sufficient fuel to sustain that energy. Exercising when you have not been eating the right foods is like putting your foot down on the accelerator and suddenly finding you have no power.

It especially important when you are putting extra demands on your body that you nourish it with the right foods. These are carbohydrates that break down slowly in the body (*see below*), such as whole grains, beans, and lentils; vegetables and fruits, which are particularly rich in phytochemicals; and protein. Water is also critical (*see pp84–85*). Dehydration can lead to muscle fatigue and loss of coordination, so it is vital when you are exercising to increase your intake to more than the recommended eight glasses of water a day.

Carbohydrates

The best fuel for sustained exercise is carbohydrates, which are broken down to glucose in the body and stored primarily in your muscles and liver as glycogen. This is then converted back into glucose to provide fuel for the muscles you are exercising. The body can only store a certain amount of glycogen, and it cannot be transferred from resting muscles to those that are working, so the glycogen in the muscles you use as you power walk will become depleted quite rapidly. Consequently, it is important to keep your levels topped off, and to have a carbohydrate snack immediately after exercise to speed recovery.

Although all carbohydrates are converted to glucose in the body, the rate at which they are absorbed differs widely. Foods such as beans, legumes, and whole grains are absorbed slowly and will provide fuel over the longer term, making them ideal foods if you are going to undertake strenuous exercise.

A green approach

Studies have consistently shown that people who eat a vegetarian diet live longer than meat-eaters and have lower incidences of many major diseases, including cancer, heart disease, and diabetes. Yet many people have concerns about meeting all their nutritional needs through a vegetarian diet, especially when they are active in sports. It is sometimes thought, for example, that an athlete needs to dig in to a large steak to gain sufficient protein, but in fact most of us in the West consume far more protein than we need, and just a few almonds provides the protein equivalent of an average steak. We can all obtain the proteins we need from many plant foods, including soy, legumes, grains, and all nuts and seeds. A word of warning: do not replace meat with equivalent amounts of cheese, since it is high in saturated fats.

Eating a wide range of plant-based foods will provide you with a high intake of antioxidants and phytochemicals, all of which have innumerable health-giving properties. They will also provide a good source of calcium (found in, for example, raw broccoli, sunflower seeds, almonds, and Brazil nuts), which is vital for strong, healthy bones and keeping active.

Eating for a marathon

If you have been following the food guidelines and training plans set out in this book, your body will be in good shape to take on the challenge of a marathon. Even so, it is important to take care with your diet right before and right after the event.

The week before

By now, training will be minimal, which will decrease the use of glycogen. Keep your food light and simple. Eat plenty of vegetables, steamed or roasted, and include one vegetable juice or smoothie a day. Salads with light dressings, grilled fish (or very lean meat), and plenty of unrefined carbohydrates such as potatoes, rice, or quinoa are ideal. Avoid rich sauces, spicy dishes, fried foods, big meals that are heavy to digest, and alcohol, which is dehydrating. Eat every 2–3 hours, using cereal bars as snacks. Also, drink plenty of water, so that on the day of the event you are well hydrated and need only sip small amounts on a regular basis.

The day before

Make sure you have two good high-carbohydrate meals. Always try to eat your largest meal in the middle of the day, so that your body does not have to work hard at digestion through the night.

The Big Day

Have a good breakfast of cereal or pancakes and fruit about 2 hours before the start. Apart from water, it is wise to take something that will give you a burst of energy, such as a banana, raisins, energy bars, or glucose tablets. Do not try any unfamiliar foods or you may end up with an upset stomach. You should also avoid anything salty or dry, such as nuts.

Immediately after the event, eat a carbohydrate snack such as a sandwich or muffin to aid your recovery, and choose a carbohydrate-led meal for the post-event dinner.

ENERGY-BOOSTING FOODS

Brown rice Unrefined brown long-grain rice is a complex carbohydrate with twice the fiber and nutrients of white rice. It is the best rice for slow absorption. As well as being a good source of protein, it also contains zinc, magnesium, vitamin B6, and selenium.

Bananas They are one of the richest sources of potassium, which helps to regulate muscle contractions. Bananas will replenish the potassium lost through sweating and are therefore an ideal snack when you are exercising strenuously.

Broccoli This is high in fiber and a good source of iron and folic acid. Iron helps to bind oxygen in red blood cells, which is then transported and used by the body's muscles, organs, and tissues. Folic acid is important for the health of red blood cells and keeping cholesterol levels under control. If eaten raw, broccoli also provides calcium.

Beans and legumes Dried beans, peas, and lentils make superb low-burning foods that are also high in protein and are a good source of folic acid (see *Broccoli, above*).

Carrot juice When freshly juiced (see *p89*) it is a concentrated source of vitamin A (beta-carotene), which is essential for the growth and repair of body tissues, and will help to fight infections.

Dried fruits These are an excellent concentrated source of energy and are rich in iron (see *Broccoli, above*) and calcium. They are high in fructose and very sweet, but they make a good snack to put in your fanny pack.

Papaya This exotic fruit has as much potassium as bananas (see *Bananas, above*), as well as high levels of vitamin C and beta-carotene (see *Carrot juice, above*).

Pasta Choose whole-wheat or buckwheat pasta when you are looking for slow-burning fuel for your muscles. A pasta dish is the perfect pre-marathon meal. Pasta also provides iron and the B vitamins thiamine, niacin, and riboflavin.

Potatoes A medium-sized portion of this powerhouse vegetable provides twice the potassium of a banana (see *Bananas, above*), and is high in vitamin C and iron (see *Broccoli, above*). They are excellent for boosting blood energy levels and fighting fatigue.

WALKING FOR YOU

Whether your main objective is to raise money for charity, care for your body during pregnancy, lose a little weight, or just have fun days out with your family, walking has the answer. It is one of the easiest and simplest ways in which you can bring fitness into every day of your life, regardless of age or ability.

[Walking is] "a delectable madness, very good for sanity." COLIN FLETCHER

FIT WALKING INTO YOUR DAY

Most of us live busy lives, our days filled to the brim. How, we ask ourselves, can we possibly squeeze in one more activity? With power walking the answer is, very easily. You can slot in a walk at any time that suits you, and it can be as long or as short as you want it to be. Once you are committed to a regular walking program, you may be surprised to find that you have more energy and greater mental clarity, and that you are more productive and use your time more efficiently.

How many times have you promised yourself that you will visit the gym, or start a fitness regimen, but failed because you put other things first, leaving no time to stick to those good intentions? Usually, work, children, or other commitments come first, leaving little time left for us to spend on ourselves. Yet if a friend asks for a favor, we usually find time to help. So why are we never that kind to ourselves?

Many of us expend much of our energy on others, both physically and emotionally. There is nothing wrong with doing this, as long as we make time for our own needs, too, such as hobbies, pampering, and exercise. Walking is one of the easiest, most accessible, and rewarding ways of giving back to ourselves. You can do it anywhere, and you don't need anyone else. The rewards come fast, and there are no rules governing how long you do it for and when, because even a short walk will have an impact. You also don't have to rely on a club or gym. Walking fulfills all the essential criteria for a busy person.

In truth, we can all find the time to do something if it is important enough to us. The secret to fitting walking into your life is to change your perspective on how you spend your time and to accept the value of allocating time for yourself.

Be realistic

With many things in life, it is far better to go for quality rather than quantity. The amount of time you dedicate to your health and fitness is no exception. Be selective with your time, and be thoughtful about choosing how, and when, you spend the time you have set aside for yourself. The greater enjoyment you receive while walking, the more you will benefit from it. There is little point in striding out for an hour, only to feel guilty and stressed on your return because there were other things you should have been doing. It is better to be realistic, walk for less time, and be able to leave all your concerns behind.

Apply time-management skills, prioritize the tasks in your day, and learn how to say no, and you will notice a big difference. We often waste precious time being overwhelmed and stressed, rather than calmly deciding on a plan. As a starting point, try to find 30 minutes for walking, preferably at the same time each day, and make that time sacrosanct. You will soon be guarding the time jealously, and everyone else will accept it as part of your routine. To find the time, you could walk the children to school instead of driving, walk to an appointment, get off the bus or train a stop earlier than usual and walk the rest of the way to work, or even get up half an hour earlier in the morning. You decide when you take the 30 minutes, but make sure you always do it.

Be prepared

Have a selection of different routes planned and ready (*see pp38–39*), including a short route for days when you have only 15–20 minutes free. Try to plot some of the routes through a park or woods, so you can spend time within a calming atmosphere and remove yourself from everything. Also plot a route near work so that you won't need to spend time wondering where to go if you find time to walk during your lunch break. Keep a second set of gear at work so that there really are no excuses for missing a chance to walk.

Book an appointment

One way to create time for walking is to write in walking sessions on your calendar. If each walking appointment is blocked out in pen, you can make other commitments work around them, and only

FINDING TIME TO WALK

Less is more: a short walk may be more enjoyable and fun than a long walk that takes up too much of your time and leaves you feeling stressed and under pressure.

Be creative with your time, and walk part or all of the way when you would otherwise drive.

Be prepared by arranging some walking routes. A variety of walks is a big key to motivation.

Make an appointment with yourself for a walking date and stick to it; learn how to say no to others.

Join a walking group, form one of your own, or find a walking buddy; shared activities are more inspiring.

reluctantly should you have to give up your walking times. You can tell people that you have an appointment at that time, but you don't need to say what it is for. Your 30 minutes of walking might not sound that important to them, and you could find yourself being persuaded to alter your plans. Doing this will also raise your awareness of any other spaces in your week when you could take additional time for yourself.

Get some allies

One of the best ways to fit walking into your schedule is to join a walking group (*see p97*). You could join one that exists locally, or even form a group of your own. Group members will encourage you to show up, which will motivate you to attend regularly. Alternatively, try to find a like-minded person who has a lifestyle similar to yours. If you have children, perhaps a shared babysitter will solve the problem of time. If you work shifts, maybe you can meet others who want to walk late at night. Make a walk a social event, work together on a training plan, and set up a regular time and place to meet.

ONE, TWO, THREE OR MORE

Power walking is a sport that works whether you want to train on your own, with a friend, or as part of a group. If you have a busy, demanding life, walking alone may give you precious breathing space. On the other hand, time spent power walking with a friend is always filled with fun, motivation, and good conversation. Joining a walking group is a popular way to combine walking with a social life.

Going solo

Walking alone is one of the greatest pleasures of power walking. With no one else to consider, you can test your personal best time, walking at top speed to your own rhythm, and feel the power and exhilaration of using your body. I relish an unaccompanied walk when I want to let off steam at the end of a busy day, or if I'm building up speed for a marathon.

If you have a problem to solve, going for a solitary walk provides you with the perfect opportunity to think things through without any distractions. Your body can pound along on automatic pilot, leaving your mind free to ponder. I usually find that after about half an hour of turning over an issue in my mind, I almost always have a solution to my worry.

Many people find that walking alone is conducive to creative thinking. Before you set off, prime your mind to focus on a given subject, but as you start walking, switch your attention to your surroundings. Let your senses open to everything around you: people, buildings, animals, flowers, trees. Keep a steady, easy pace, don't try to force inspirational thoughts, but trust that they will float up from your unconscious to your conscious mind, naturally and effortlessly. Take a small notepad and pen in your walk bag so that you can jot down your thoughts. A variation on this theme is to mindful walking (*see pp82–83*).

Make sure when you are walking alone that you pick routes where you feel safe from traffic or people (*see also pp116–117*).

Tête-à-tête

Walking with a friend will often get you out of the door when you lack the drive to do it yourself, and will ensure that you walk regularly and more often. Plan routes and training programs together so that you are both equally involved. Take turns acting as the pacesetter so that you don't reach a fitness plateau. Working at improving your fitness also gives added purpose to your walks.

Talking while you are walking makes the time fly by, and it is a good benchmark for exertion (*see also pp34–37*). If you are able to carry on a conversation with no difficulty, then your pace may be too easy. At a moderate to high-intensity pace, you should be able to keep talking, but you may be slightly breathless. If the talking stops and you are out of breath, then you are pushing yourself too hard and should slow down.

WALKING FOR ONE

Plan your walking routes carefully when walking alone to be sure you do not stray into an unsafe neighborhood. Take all the usual safety precautions and always let somebody know where you are going. Walking alone can be an inspiring, empowering experience, but it is no fun if you do not feel safe.

Part of the crowd

Apart from the camaraderie that a walking group brings, it also provides a constant source of encouragement and support, and a steady flow of banter and laughter. The feeling of belonging and having a common purpose that comes with being part of a group is irreplaceable. Meetings offer a social occasion, a chance to meet like-minded people, and often the means to form lasting friendships. Invariably, the larger the group, the more mixed the abilities will be. Try to pair up with those of a similar walking ability or a little better than you, which may mean splitting the group into a number of smaller groups. If this happens, arrange meeting points to regroup.

Walking groups are usually informal affairs, arranged between friends or work colleagues. However, more formal walking groups and walking clubs do exist, and you may find notices about meetings for these at your local gym or YMCA or in your local newspaper. Most clubs charge a small fee for membership to cover administration costs.

Walking with a friend is a great way to stay motivated and stick to a training program. It can also turn exercising into a social occasion.

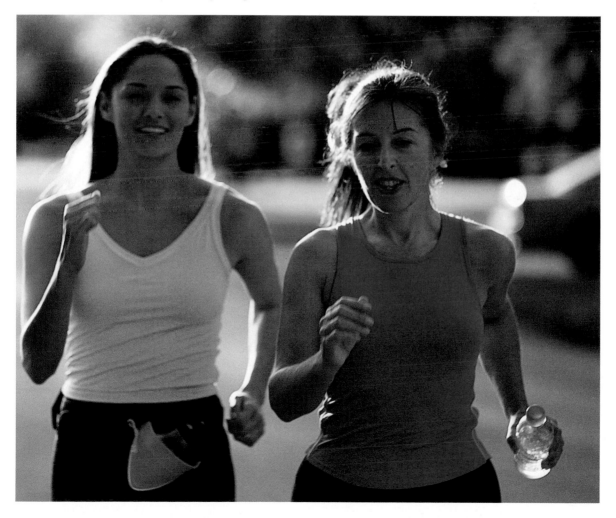

WALKING TO LOSE WEIGHT

If the average person power walks four times a week, for 45 minutes each time, he or she will lose approximately 18 lb (8kg) within a year, without changing his or her diet in any way. Add to this program regular stretching and strengthening workouts, together with a healthy, weight-aware diet, and you will have the tools you need to reach your ideal weight and feel fantastic, too.

Keep a diary

Whether your goal is to lose 5 lb (2kg) or 50 lb (22kg), there are three promises that you must make to yourself to reach your target. The first is to keep a diary. For the first week, simply write down everything you eat without making any changes to your diet. For the following three weeks, use your diary to chart what you eat, how much, and when; how far and how fast you walk; and how you feel. You must be completely honest with yourself, and include every detail, no matter how small. By doing this you can build a realistic picture of your weaknesses and strengths, and can act accordingly.

Note in your diary your ideal, and realistically achievable, weight for a month's time. Aim to lose 1–2 lb (0.5–1kg) a week on average—any more than this and you are losing water and muscle, not fat. Don't be disheartened if your weight loss is slow at the beginning of a diet. This is normal, especially when teamed with exercise, since this builds muscle, and muscle tissue weighs more than fat. How well your clothes fit can act as a good guide to weight loss. Weigh yourself once a week only, at the same time, since your weight can fluctuate on a daily basis.

Power walking burns calories efficiently, and will tone and shape your body. Eat a wide variety of healthy foods, but watch quantities when you are trying to lose weight. Keeping a diary can help you discover if you are overeating and why, and chart the success of your exercise plan.

Get moving

The second promise you need to make is to start exercising. The principle is simple: exercise aerobically to burn calories and you will lose weight, even without changing your diet. Power walking is a low-impact, aerobic exercise that burns about 300 calories an hour for the average person weighing 150 lb (70kg) and walking at a brisk pace. (The faster you walk, or the heavier you are, the more calories you will burn.) Power walking also builds muscles, and the more muscle mass you have in proportion to fat, the faster your metabolism works. Your metabolic rate is the speed at which your body naturally burns calories (energy), even when sleeping. So not only will you

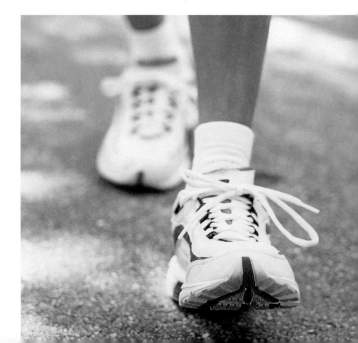

lose body fat by walking, but you will also develop the muscle that will keep it off.

For weight loss, it is recommended that you take 10,000 steps a day, of which 4,000–6,000 steps should be uninterrupted walking. Use a pedometer to record the number of steps you take and count the number of calories burned (*see pp36–37*). A heart-rate monitor (*see pp32–35*) will ensure that you raise your heart rate sufficiently to burn fat. Use the Weight Loss Program (*see pp176–181*) as a guide for your walking routine, which includes stretching and strengthening routines.

Healthy foods

The third promise is to start making healthy changes to the way you eat. I don't personally advocate any of the quick-fix diets, because they generally give short-term results and deny your body the full range of foods it needs to stay strong and vibrant.

It may be that you don't need to go on a food-reduction regimen at all. For one week, make no alterations to your diet, but write down daily everything you eat to give you an idea of your normal intake, and make a note of your walks.

At the end of the week, you may find that power walking alone is starting to give you the improved body shape you were hoping for, and you don't need to watch the amount of food you are eating. However, you may still need to make changes to the types of foods that you eat. For example, slowly replace any refined, highly processed foods with healthy alternatives, such as brown rice or pasta instead of white, and include more vegetables, whole grains, and legumes in your diet.

Even if you need to reduce portion sizes, always eat breakfast to give your metabolism a kick-start. Eat five to six small meals a day to keep your energy levels up and your metabolism steady, and to help avoid hunger pangs. Drink plenty of water (*see pp84–85*). Dehydration can give the illusion of hunger instead of thirst, and can be a cause of weight gain. Plan ahead what you will eat each day, keep an eye on fat and sugar content, and chew your food thoroughly. Don't deny yourself treats, but save them for special occasions. The success of a weight-loss plan depends on your being aware of what you are eating, making the right choices, and taking small steps to success.

WALKING AND PREGNANCY

Staying fit and healthy throughout pregnancy will give you much-needed energy and help you to feel less tired. Walking is a low-impact, noncontact form of cardiovascular exercise that you can continue doing right into the later stages of pregnancy. It will keep your muscles strong and flexible, which is invaluable during both pregnancy and labor.

If you are already a walker, continue but walk less intensively, even in the first few months. You should always discuss exercise with your doctor first in case of complications. If you are new to walking and were fairly inactive before you became pregnant, again, consult your doctor—if you are out of shape, this is not the time to start an exercise program. This is especially important in the first trimester, when you may feel super-charged with energy. Try to walk three times a week, and build up to 20–30-minute sessions.

Keep in tune with your body, and if you feel overtired, short of breath, or uncomfortable, stop immediately. Keep your walking routes close to your home and amenities, in case you get tired. Drink water before, during, and after your walk.

Alter your technique
Walking during pregnancy requires some adjustments to your technique. During and just after pregnancy your body releases the hormone relaxin, which softens and loosens your joints in preparation for childbirth. This new-found flexibility can lead to overextending in stretches and in other activities if you are not careful. It may sound wonderful to be so agile, but be cautious to avoid injury, and don't push your body too far.

During pregnancy, walk with a shorter stride than usual to create a less aggressive movement in your hips. Make sure your workout is low-impact by keeping your feet low to the ground as you walk. Note that marathons are not recommended for women at any stage of pregnancy.

Walking by trimester
In the first trimester (weeks 1–13), you can more or less follow your normal walking routine, but start to reduce the level of intensity. Don't walk in hot and humid weather, since studies indicate that overheating may cause birth defects.

In the second trimester (weeks 14–26), to avoid straining your back, watch your posture (*see pp40–41*), and remember to look ahead. Don't walk on uneven ground, such as trails and beaches—stick to pavement. Check in the second and third trimesters that your shoes are supporting your arches, which will be under pressure as your weight increases. Your feet may also swell to the point where you need shoes in the next size up.

In the third trimester (weeks 27–40), keep going for as long as you can. You will need to slow down; don't push yourself to walk farther than you feel comfortable with.

WALKING WITH YOUR BABY

About 4–6 weeks after the birth, you should be able to resume walking. You might like to carry your baby with you in a carrier or use an all-terrain stroller, but be aware of your posture. Keep your arms bent and push with your body weight, not just your shoulders. For an older baby or young child use a well-fitting backpack or carrier as it is better for your posture and technique.

THE RAISED CAT STRETCH

This stretch is based on a yoga pose and is perfect for stretching your lower back and strengthening your legs without putting any strain on the abdomen. It develops balance and focus, and has the effect of making you feel powerful and strong. Use it to replace the full-body stretches on pp66–67.

1 Begin by kneeling with hands below shoulders and knees below hips. Keep arms straight, but without locking the elbows, and eyes looking down. Make sure you are comfortable in this start position.

2 Inhale and slowly lift your right leg up and out behind you, pointing your toe and raising your head at the same time. Feel it work the back of the leg and notice the stretch along your spine.

3 Now bend your right leg and point your toe. Exhale slowly and hold the position for a few seconds. Inhale and lower your leg, returning to the start position in Step 1. Repeat on the other side. Once you are familiar with the sequence, steps 2 and 3 can be completed in one fluid movement.

WALKING WITH CHILDREN

Physical activity is essential to a child's healthy development. The earlier you can introduce regular exercise into your child's life, the greater the chance that he or she will carry this pattern through into adulthood. Walking—whether power walking or simply brisk walking—with children is a great way to get them moving. You will provide them with an important role model, and firmly implant the idea that walking is a natural and normal activity.

Statistics show that children in the developed world are becoming more sedentary, overweight, and out of shape. Fewer sports are played at school, and more time is spent in front of televisions and computers. Physical activity patterns are established in childhood, so it is vital that parents, along with schools, encourage children to get moving. Current recommendations are that they should do at least 30 minutes of moderate-intensity physical activity each day, such as playing outdoors, dancing, playing ball games, bicycling, helping with physical chores such as gardening, and, of course, walking. These activities allow children to learn motor skills, develop fitness, and increase energy expenditure, and also enhance academic performance and mental health. Start walking with children as early as possible, even if it means carrying them in the first year or so (*see pp100–101*).

In addition to walking, introduce as many fun exercise activities as possible that will encourage children to move their bodies and develop their motor skills.

WALKING TO SCHOOL

Physical activity early in the day clears away the cobwebs, and will make you and your child alert and ready to face your day. It may not be possible to walk your child to school, especially if the journey is long, but if you can, it is also a great way of spending special time with your child. If you find it more convenient, you may be able to organize a walking rotation with other parents, and take turns supervising a group walk to school.

At some point, your child may ask to be allowed to walk to school alone. Never allow him or her to walk a route you haven't checked out together with your child first, and that you have established is a safe one. Time the journey so you know how long it should take your child to get home. Always make sure that he or she has a walking buddy there and back, or better still, walks with a group of children. Walking safely is essential.

Make walking fun

Set aside regular times for walking, for 30 minutes to an hour, at least once a week if your child is already fairly physically active, and up to three or more times a week if your child is turning into a couch potato. Most children between three and seven years will make good walking companions. If you power walk, albeit at a slower pace, so will they. As a rough guide to how far you can walk with small children, estimate ½ mile (1km) per birthday. This means a three-year-old should be able to walk 2 miles (3km) in total, but allow for plenty of rests, and accept that some children are more physical and stronger than others.

Children will walk farther when there is something to see and do along the way, so try different routes (*see pp38–39*) that take in, for example, parks, streams, and woods. You may want to collect interesting things along the way, or play "I Spy." Plan your turnaround point at a playground, or even a toy shop. If children associate walking with fun activities, they will want to go again. Always remember to carry extra water for your children.

For older children, devise routes that require simple map-reading. They will love to be in charge of where to go next, and you can teach them a useful life skill at the same time. Gadgets are usually a source of fascination, so walking with a pedometer is sure to appeal. Keep a chart at home where they can record their progress, and add a reward system of stars if you wish.

Walking events

Most children enjoy noncompetitive walking events, especially if it means coming home with a medal or a T-shirt. Many charity walking events are ideal for families and are a way to share your hobby with your children. They will especially enjoy raising money for others, so try to ensure that they are sponsored, however small the final sum.

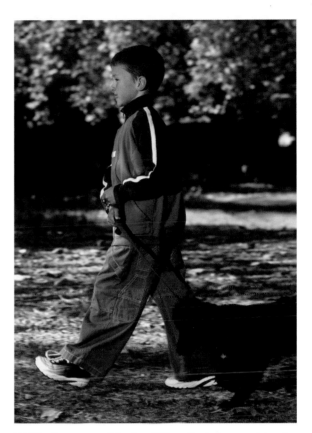

Walking is a great activity for children. Exploring a variety of surroundings in different weather conditions is a fun way to keep them interested and active, while spending time together.

Tuning into teenagers

Walking is an ideal way for teenagers to control their weight healthily and sensibly. Teenagers need challenges, so activities such as hiking (*see pp112–113*) or orienteering are good ways to keep them active. Orienteering is a sport that involves quickly navigating your way between designated control points marked on a map. It is a great way to explore the countryside, and can be quite physical, depending on the terrain. Check to see if there is an orienteering club in your area that organizes a range of events.

Walking events and marathons often have an under-17 category. These tend to be popular and well attended.

WALKING FOR CHARITIES

A rewarding and positive way to create an incentive to get fitter, as well as set a personal goal, is to take part in a walking challenge. By entering a charity challenge, you will experience the wonderful camaraderie of many like-minded people raising money and awareness for a worthy cause. There are a multitude of causes, from environment and wildlife, to child welfare, to disease, and many others. There will almost certainly be an event near you that suits your ability and concern.

For first-timers

If you have a favorite cause or charity, find out if they are involved with any walking events and what distances they include. There are many sponsored walks and challenges that you can take part in, and whether it is in your local community or a national event, all charities will welcome you to their team.

Make sure that you are prepared to commit to the required training before signing up to the event. For the short-distance walker, beginners, or those wanting a less demanding challenge, there are plenty of 3-mile (5km) and 6-mile (10km) walks, which are ideal distances. Depending on your

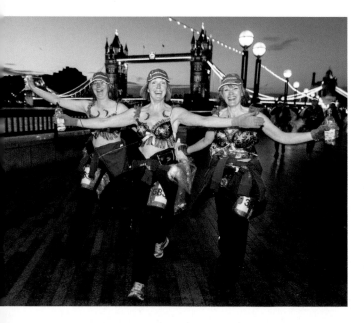

starting fitness, preparation may take only three or four weeks, while a full marathon, for example, will require around three months of training. Browse pp140–187 for guidance on what training you can expect for different distances.

Before making a commitment to any challenge, check the closing time of the finish line, as it can be different in every case. Some running marathons that also accept walkers will close within 6–7 hours. This makes proper training essential, as this will be the time you have to complete the distance to ensure you receive your medal. However, other events may not be so demanding and are geared more toward mixed abilities and families. At this point, you might also want to consider whether you would rather walk alone and set a personal goal, or walk with a group. Training with others is not only sociable, it is often the source of many friendships. The team spirit means that motivation and encouragement are always on hand when you need it most.

Sponsorship and fundraising

With popular events, the demand to enter can far outweigh the availability of places. Charities often have their own entry allocations. These are

Walk the Walk organises the iconic MoonWalk in major cites, such as London. All the walkers wear a trademark decorated bra to raise money and awareness for breast cancer.

available to anyone provided you are willing to commit to raising a specified minimum amount of sponsorship money for that charity. Before you enter, it is important to think about whether or not you will be able to easily raise the funds required. In some cases, the amount can be quite high, so not meeting the level of funds required could mean the charity loses money. Maximize your ability to raise your sponsorship by using online fundraising. Your chosen charity will be able to help and advise you with plenty of inspirational ideas and suggestions on how to increase your fundraising.

Expand your horizons

If you have completed a shorter distance and enjoyed the experience, expand your horizons and try a 10-mile (16km) event, a half-marathon (13 miles/21km), a full marathon (26¼ miles/42.2km), or even an ultra-distance, such as 62 miles (100km).

Taking on a challenge that involves travelling to another country will undoubtedly add a new level of excitement to your adventure. If you are not tied to a specific cause, search for a charity that offers to refund your traveling expenses. (This will be subject to you raising a specified amount.) The result is a great exchange because you get to travel, and the charity receives much-needed funds. For those who want to push themselves to the next level, there is plenty to choose from. Classic marathons include cities such as New York, Paris, or Berlin, or even walking the Great Wall of China. There are now also quite a number of 100-mile (161km) events, including the historic four-day Nijmegen Marches in the Netherlands. Some of these events can be primarily for runners, so check that as a walker you meet their conditions. Once you have entered any challenge, carefully read through the information that is sent to you and make a point of noting any important details that will be relevant on the day, especially where you

The start line of a marathon is always very exciting. Crowds and supporters can really help to motivate you. Write your name on your T-shirt so that they can cheer you on.

will find the information point, water, toilets, and first aid stop.

Walk the Walk, the charity I founded, specializes in organizing a wide range of power walking challenges within the UK and around the world. It raises money for vital breast cancer causes and promotes walking as an important part of good health and cancer prevention. Challenges include 3 miles (5km), to multi-marathons, to trekking in Peru, to even an Arctic experience. Our famous MoonWalks that see thousands power walking a marathon through the night are held in cities such as London and New York. Check our program pages for guidance on training schedules (see pp140–187).

COMPETITIVE WALKING

Entering a competitive event is an excellent way to keep you motivated and focused. Make sure that you set yourself a challenging, but achievable, goal; no matter how many times you have raced, it is always exciting to cross the finish line to receive your medal. If you are a fast power walker and you would like to push yourself a bit further, discover a different type of challenge altogether with either speed walking or racewalking.

Most competitive races take place on roads and are primarily for runners, but these are still ideal for power walkers to take part in. Some marathons now even offer a walkers category. Often a fit and fast power walker will match the pace of a runner, so don't be discouraged from entering. However, it is important never to accidentally block in a runner and prevent him or her from passing.

Road races are fun events, and many double as money-raisers for charity (*see pp104–105*), although some people will be taking part simply to win or gain a good recorded time. There are many

Racewalking is the recognized sport for walkers. It is a sociable sport with clubs worldwide that organize races over a range of distances.

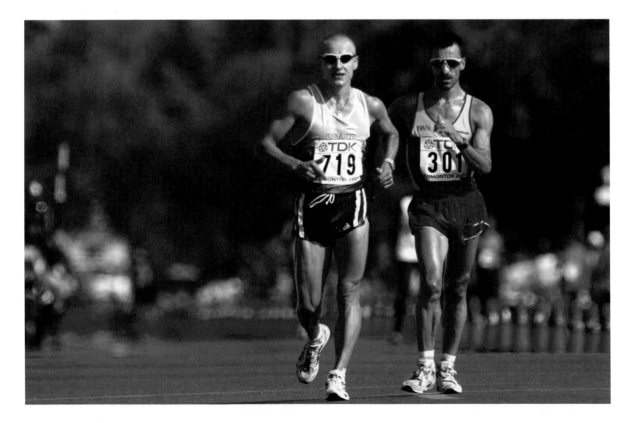

NO LAST-MINUTE CHANGES

Many people make the mistake of wearing new clothing or, even worse, new walking shoes on the day of their marathon or competition walk. My advice is to keep everything exactly the same on that day as it has been in training, including your clothes and equipment, so that you won't get any surprises. Shoes in particular need to be worn in to ensure minimal blisters.

different lengths of races available, so you can start with a shorter distance and build up to a marathon over time.

Entering a marathon

Never underestimate the training needed to be sure you finish a marathon. A marathon is 26¼ miles (42.2km) long, and can take, on average, between 5 and 10 hours to complete, which is a significant amount of time to be on your feet. You should allow yourself a minimum of three months to prepare, particularly if you are aiming for a good finishing time. If you have never walked before, you will need to allow longer to train, anything from 12 to 18 weeks. You will find a full training program for walking a marathon on pp170–175.

Fifty percent of walking a successful marathon is in your mind and the belief that you can accomplish it. Depending on your level of fitness and power-walking ability, your aim should be to walk at a fast and constantly maintained pace over the entire distance. You will also need to modify your diet toward the end of your training. For advice on what you need to eat and drink on the days leading up to the marathon, see pp90–91. On the day, wear your usual training clothes (*see also box, top*). Comfortable feet are vital to your performance (*see pp18–23*). Slather your feet with petroleum jelly, since this is an excellent way to prevent blisters (*see also p128*).

Speed walking and racewalking

When you reach a consistent walking pace of 5 mph (8km/h) or more, you naturally feel that you want to start running. This is because running is the easier way to move comfortably at high speed initially, and it is also your body's natural energy-saving option. However, if you do continue walking instead and push the body a little more intensely, you will find that you are speed walking. Speed walking is a milder, slower form of racewalking, just the same as jogging is to running. Interestingly, both speed walking and racewalking use more energy and burn more calories mile for mile than running. It is relatively easy to progress from power and speed walking to racewalking, but it will help if you can join a club to receive coaching on the racewalking technique. (*See pp170–175 for a full marathon training plan*).

There are two main rules in racewalking that must be strictly adhered to. First, a walker must maintain contact with the ground at all times. This means that the leading foot must be planted before lifting the back foot. Second, the knee of the leading leg must be kept straight from the moment each foot touches the ground until the leg is vertical. These restrictions result in your hips rotating as your weight shifts from side to side, and consequently gives racewalkers their unique wiggle.

Racewalking is an endurance sport but, like power walking, it has the benefit of being low-impact and therefore has a low risk of injury. It is a very sociable sport with clubs all over the world. Members are always eager to enlist new walkers and very willing to help all levels and ages of newcomers.

Racewalking is a major sport and is represented in the Olympic and Commonwealth games. Clubs will cover distances from 1 mile (1.6 km) to 100 miles (161km) or more.

OUT AND ABOUT

You can power walk almost anywhere, at any time, which makes power walking one of the most accessible ways to keep fit. Even extreme weather need not be a deterrent, as long as you have the right clothing and equipment for the conditions. Try combining road walking with hill walking and include other types of terrain for some of your walks. These will not only challenge you physically, the variety in your walks will also keep you motivated.

"An early-morning walk is a blessing for the whole day."
HENRY DAVID THOREAU

ROAD WALKING

Roads and pavements are easily accessible for walkers. The advantage of walking on asphalt or paving is that the surface is generally flat and even, which means less strain is placed on ankles and knees, so the risk of injury is reduced. Road walking is particularly good for interval training. While it is possible to interval train on any surface or terrain, the more even the ground, the greater the opportunity to concentrate on your speed and technique.

If you are considering taking part in a long-distance walking event, you will need to have experienced training on asphalt because most events will take place on roads. As part of your training, you may want to introduce interval training, which will help to increase your fitness levels.

Interval training

Your heart is a muscle that needs to be trained like any other, and this is what interval training is designed specifically to do. The training involves alternately walking for periods of time at a high intensity (faster) and periods of low intensity (slower). This increases your fitness and aerobic strength and stamina. The periods of intense walking should feel like all-out exertion, and the slower periods are designed for you to recover your breath and composure ready to repeat another interval of intensity.

Interval training is extremely effective at burning fat. The harder periods will work your body at a high level that raises your metabolic rate (see pp98–99) enough to continue burning fat (calories) for up to 18 hours after your walk.

Begin as you would for any walk by warming up and stretching (see pp68–72). Once you are warm

Walking on roads and pavement prepares you for long-distance events and is the perfect surface for interval training, a fat-burning, high-intensity aerobic cardio workout.

and have a good flow to your walk you can begin interval training. The length and intensity of both the fast and slow intervals will depend on your level of fitness. The extra stress put on your heart through this training means it is not ideal for someone with a low level of fitness, so check with your doctor to determine if it is suitable for you.

The intervals at a faster speed should be short bursts and can last from 30 seconds to 3 minutes. The slower-speed intervals are longer and can last 2–15 minutes. As a guide, start with a ratio of 1:2, so for every 1 minute walked at an intense, fast pace, you should double it for the slow, recovery pace. If it feels too tough or too easy, adjust the length of intervals accordingly. As your fitness improves, try a ratio of 1:1, so that the periods of fast and slow walking are equal in length.

Each of your fast and slow periods should be of a similar intensity throughout the whole walk. Don't start with a pace so fast you won't be able to repeat it at each interval. Complete your session as you would any walk by cooling down and stretching (see pp68–72). Interval training is challenging and should be limited to a couple of times a week. You will find it beneficial to keep a log to monitor your progress in interval training.

A treadmill (see pp136–137) is useful for interval training because accurate monitoring of the length and speed of each interval is easy. Treadmills are sprung, so softer to walk on than other terrains.

TRAIL WALKING

Walking on trails in different terrains can be a pleasant change from road walking. In particular, conquering hills is a great way to increase the intensity of your walk, improve your endurance levels, and burn more calories. You will also test your core stability when covering uneven ground. To get the full enjoyment and benefit of this type of walking, you will need to make changes to both your technique and your clothing.

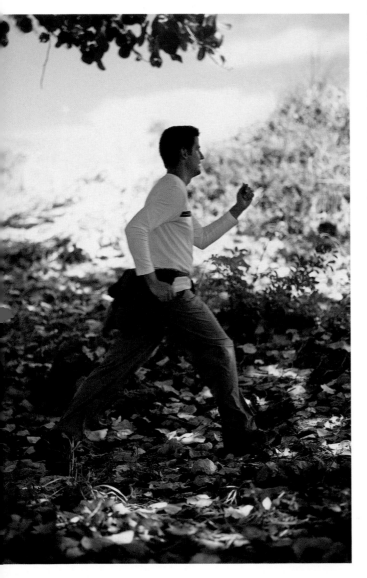

The most demanding part of trail walking is usually navigating hills, and you will need to prepare for this. Approach hill training in the same way as road walking, by starting slowly with short walks and building up from there. Begin by including more hills in your road power-walking routes or increasing the incline on your treadmill a little. Over a period of about two weeks or so, your legs should become accustomed to the change of angle. Unfortunately, there is no easy way to prepare your body for walking downhill, and consequently even strong walkers are sometimes surprised by how difficult they find it.

Changes in your technique

To assist you in walking up a hill, shorten your step to use your body more efficiently and lean forward slightly as the incline becomes more acute. To descend, again, keep your stride short and lean back a little, but not too far. Going down a hill sounds easy, but this is just as challenging as going up because the impact of your body weight increases from 1½ times your normal weight to 5 times your normal weight. This puts extra stress on your limbs and joints, and to begin with, you may even find it a little painful.

Walking on rough ground can work out different parts of your body. On uneven surfaces, you will need to consider a change in your shoes and clothing.

NORDIC WALKING

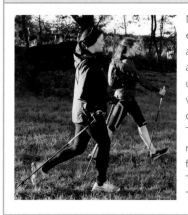

Nordic walking is a cardiovascular and endurance activity. It appeals to all abilities, not just avid walkers looking for a new experience. It is also extensively used by those who are restricted from walking without support due to medical conditions, or rehabilitating from an injury. The exertion level can be as vigorous as required, and you can walk anywhere, from city pavements to country fields. The only essential equipment is the poles. These must be the correct type and length to allow fluid movement, as they become an extension of your body. By using a specific technique, aided by a hand grip that is attached to the pole, weight is taken off the knees and lower body joints. This increases upper-body and core use, making it feel easier to move faster than normal walking, so you can walk farther and for longer. Initially, it is advisable to join a local group, to get the benefit of coaching on the correct technique and to meet other walkers.

Your ankles, knees, hips, and lower back will all help to stabilize you and will take the strain of walking on uneven ground. Your outer thigh muscles (abductors) in particular will be working much harder than usual. Focus on strengthening the muscles in these areas and your core stability muscles to give you maximum support (*see pp54–59*).

Clothes and useful extras

Your shoes are key to your overall comfort, particularly if you are going to be walking at awkward angles on uneven terrain for continuous periods of time. When walking off-road, it is better to wear a shoe that is durable and has deep treads for good traction. A Gore-Tex shoe is very light, protective, and waterproof. Allow ample room for your toes, because your foot will slide forward in your shoe as you walk downhill.

For rugged trails and walking in winter, wear a rigid, waterproof hiking boot that covers your ankle to give maximum protection and support so your ankles and knees don't twist. Whatever your footwear, get used to it—its weight, and the way your foot moves inside it—before going out on a long walk.

Where the hikes are less challenging, you can wear the same clothes as for power walking (*see pp24–25*). However, you may want to substitute lightweight walking pants or a pair of shorts for your leggings. When you are walking in hills, a warm sunny day can become cold and wet very quickly, so be prepared with a windproof jacket, a fleece, and waterproof clothing. With more extreme conditions, it is advisable to get expert advice on specific equipment (*see also pp114–115*).

When out for the day, take a small backpack rather than a fanny pack, which may be too small to carry everything you need. Practice walking with a backpack on your back for a few flat road walks first to get used to the weight. You will need plenty of water, some food, insect repellent, waterproof clothing, a detailed map of the area, the safety items on p116, and a compass. It is important that you are able to read a map and understand the symbols before setting out.

Walking poles can be useful on rough or steep ground. They come in varying weights, and today some are surprisingly light. The poles are most useful to aid your balance, particularly on a descent.

Finally, a note on safety. As trail walking becomes better known, it is probably wise not to walk alone. Go with a friend or join a group.

WALKING IN DIFFERENT CLIMATES

Extreme weather can be a challenge, but rarely are the conditions so bad that you need be prevented from enjoying your walk. Heading out on crisp new snow or with the sun warming your skin can be a great experience. For a walk to be a success in extreme heat or cold, it is important to be prepared by wearing the correct clothing, knowing your limitations, and learning all you can to make yourself safe and comfortable.

Always check the weather forecast so that you can decide if a walk is possible that day and prepare for the conditions. Even the most physically fit person will have days when a walk is out of the question. Note that temperatures above 95°F (35°C) or below −10°F (−23°C) are always unsafe.

When walking in extreme heat, be cautious and slow your pace down if the temperature is above 80°F (26°C). Also check the heat index. High humidity can push the apparent temperature up by as much as 10°F (5°C) because the moisture in the air prevents your sweat from evaporating, and it is this evaporation that cools you. Heat stroke and heat exhaustion can be very serious. To avoid suffering from either, walk at the coolest times of day, before 11:00 a.m. and after 3:00 p.m. You may need to slow your pace and keep alert to how you feel. At the first sign of dizziness or a headache, stop walking and cool down.

In the same way, be aware of the wind chill factor, which can turn a cold day into a freezing one. In cold conditions your heart has to work extra hard for you to walk and keep warm. If you have a heart problem, you should consult a doctor before walking in very cold weather. To avoid the most severe conditions, try to walk in the middle, and warmest, part of the day.

Keeping cool in the heat

When walking in heat, always drink plenty of water to stay hydrated. Your body will sweat more than in normal weather, and can need as much as double your normal intake of water to replace lost fluids. Drink 1 pint (0.5 liters) of water both before and after your walk, and drink regularly during your walk, at least every 15–20 minutes.

While preoccupied with walking, you may be unaware of the sun's intensity until it is too late. Wear light or white clothes to reflect the sun's heat, and choose those that are made from moisture-wicking fabrics. Invest in sun-protective clothes if you can; their sun protection factor (SPF) ranges from SPF 30 to SPF 100. Wear clothing that covers the body rather than exposing it. A hat is essential, preferably one that covers the back of your neck, and you should always wear UV protection sunglasses. Apply a suitable strength sunscreen

TIPS ON KEEPING COOL

Freeze half a bottle of water and top it off with cold water before you set out. You will then have a cool drink, at least until the ice melts.

For a cool head, soak an old cotton hat in cold water, and make holes in it to release the heat.

To keep your body cool, use a spray bottle filled with water to mist your walking top. The dampened material will keep you cooler for longer.

TIPS ON KEEPING WARM

Alter your stride so that your pace is shorter and quicker to raise the heart rate and keep you warm.

Always wear a hat that covers your ears—60 percent of your body heat is lost through the top of the head.

Carry a small, handheld hot pack to warm your hands if you really feel the chill.

If you have asthma, you may want to breathe warm air, so wear a scarf to cover your chin and mouth.

liberally all over, even under your clothes, then reapply later, because sweating will rub it off.

Protecting against the cold

In cold conditions it is essential to warm up and stretch thoroughly before setting out. Do your cool-down stretches indoors, and after your walk, change out of your clothes quickly to avoid getting a chill.

Wear two or three layers of thin thermal garments. These will trap warm air between the layers and keep you warm, and can be removed if you get hot. A flexible waterproof jacket with underarm and side zippers will give you the option to let your body breathe. A detachable hood with a peak is a must, with drawstrings to fit it close to your head—most ski jackets are ideal. Wear thermal long johns underneath your leggings, but nothing that restricts movement. To keep your feet dry, invest in sturdy, waterproof shoes with good treads in case the ground is treacherous. You may have to accept less flexibility in your shoes, and consequently less speed, but it means you can continue walking.

In cold weather, wearing mittens combined with a strong arm movement will help your upper body and hands to stay warm as you walk.

SAFETY

Whether you are walking in a busy city or down quiet country roads, alone or with a group, you need to be aware of walking safely. Our roads are busier than ever, and no one wants to be constantly looking over their shoulder. By using common sense combined with some practical advice, you can feel confident in the knowledge that you are well prepared and can focus on enjoying your walk.

The secret of walking safely is planning ahead. Step one: Make sure you keep a ready-packed fanny pack with all the essential items, and use a water bottle holder. Step two: Plan your route carefully. Step three: Wear high-visibility clothing both on your front and back. It doesn't matter what time of day you are walking or the weather conditions, it is important to be seen at all times. Step four: Ensure you have a fully charged phone, and that you have installed the ICE app (in case of an emergency). This will place any important medical information or contact details visibly onto the screen of a locked phone. You can also write the information in permanent ink on the inside flap of your fanny pack. Following these simple guidelines will allow you to feel more relaxed and in control.

Essentials for your fanny pack

The following list may seem like a lot of items, but it is better to be prepared for any eventuality. Choose a fanny pack that is compact, and ideally with several pockets so that you can find things easily (see also pp28–29.)

Keep a small jar of petroleum jelly to rub onto your feet in case your shoes begin to rub, and for your lips, especially in cold weather. Tissues, surgical tape for any blister-prone areas, and a few adhesive bandages are good to have for any minor injuries. Paper and a short pencil can be useful for making any notes that come to mind. (I always have my most creative thoughts while walking!) Carry enough money to buy extra water and snacks, as well as to cover the cost of a taxi or

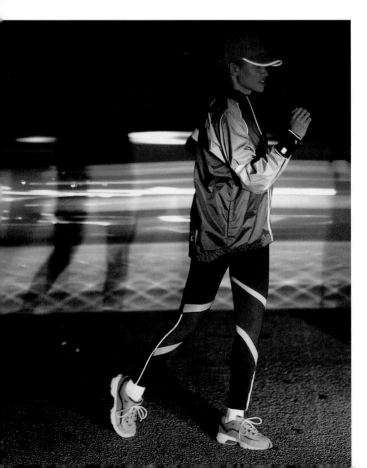

Outfit yourself for walking in the dark with reflective strips attached to your clothing, footwear, and hat. It's essential to be seen and recognized as a moving body.

transportation home if required. Add your local taxi company to your phone contacts. You may want to include a pollution mask if you regularly walk in areas of heavy traffic and want to cut down on inhaling exhaust fumes. A small personal alarm that you know how to use—and for walking at night, a headlamp—can also be useful.

Always keep your pack loaded and ready to go so that each time you walk, you only need to remember water, keys, a phone, and something to snack on (such as a banana or cereal bar).

Plan your route

There are plenty of apps that you can now download to plot and plan a variety of routes that will work alongside your fitness and training plan. When you have determined your route, always check it in daylight and by car before setting off on foot. For safety and interest, it is always a good idea to regularly change your route.

Walking in the dark

It is not enough just to wear light-colored clothes when walking at night, or when visibility is poor. High-visibility clothing helps you to be seen and recognized as a moving body. Most shoes and technical sports clothing come with reflective marks, but you can also buy separate accessories for added safety. Carry a headlamp in case you need additional light, but only choose walks that you know and that are in well-lit areas.

It can be great to walk alone, but always let somebody know where you are walking and what time you expect to return. If it is really unavoidable that your walk travels through areas you are unsure of, it is better to walk with a friend. The limited daylight hours of winter walking can be challenging, so creating your own walking group can be a good option.

CHECK LIST TO SAFETY

Carry a loaded fanny pack with all your essentials, plus a holder for your water so that your hands are kept free.

Fully charge your phone and add ICE (in case of emergency) details. But avoid using your phone to chat, or using any other electronic devices that take your attention off the road while walking. Be aware of your environment—be it a dog, cyclist, a fast car, or other people around you.

Always walk in the direction facing oncoming traffic, if your route does not have sidewalks or bike paths. Try to avoid any areas that you are unsure of.

Dress to be seen and wear reflective garments. Drivers are not expecting to see you. At the very least, wear a white T-shirt over your walking clothes.

Carrying a personal alarm can make you feel more comfortable, but make sure you know how to use it.

Always trust your instincts. If you feel uneasy at any time, breathe out slowly to help you relax and gain control. Keep moving and head for a busy area to ask for help in a store or restaurant.

Always try to look confident and aware of your surroundings. When walking toward a stranger, keep your eyes neutral. Allow your gaze to rest briefly on the person, then look to either side of them. This signals that you are not fazed by his or her presence.

Carry the number of a local taxi company and enough money for transportation home should you need it.

Enjoy planning and trying out new routes in daylight, preferably by car before starting to walk them. Download an app that allows others to track you while you are walking.

Avoid unnecessary risk and prepare. Before venturing out, ask yourself, "Who am I walking with?", "Where will I, or we, walk?", "Does somebody know where I am walking?", "Do I have everything I need?", "Do I have enough water?", and "Is my phone fully charged?" Most importantly, use your common sense and awareness to continually re-evaluate your surroundings while you are walking.

CARING FOR YOUR BODY

Regular exercise makes you feel great, but don't forget to spend a little time caring for yourself too. Treat yourself to a regular pedicure and foot massage, which will release stress, relax your body, and keep your feet in good condition. Prevent injuries by stretching and strengthening vulnerable areas, and act quickly on minor problems with home treatments that are simple but effective.

"Life is not merely being alive, but being well."

MARTIAL

BE BODY AWARE

If we take our bodies for granted, we risk ignoring the warning signals they send out in the form of aches and pains when we have overexercised or suffered an injury. In the following pages, you will learn how to diagnose, treat, and prevent some of the most common walking injuries. By listening to your body and adhering to a few rules, you should stay injury-free.

As you begin power walking, you will naturally become more aware of your body, and the effect exercise has on it, both good and bad. Pay attention to your body so that you know how it feels when it is functioning normally. You will then find it easier to recognize an imminent injury, how the stresses of your everyday life are affecting you, or if you are coming down with an ailment.

Recognizing the signs

Mild aches and pains are the body's early-warning system. Learn how to read these signs so you can decide whether it is better to rest or train that day. If something is wrong, a self-treatment at home may be all that is required, but if you are in doubt and the pain is severe or chronic, err on the side of caution and consult a doctor.

You may find that as you start power walking, it aggravates an old injury that was not treated properly at the time it occurred. Alternatively, you may discover that you have uncovered a muscular or postural imbalance that was not evident before. In either of these instances, discuss the problem with your doctor.

A useful way of keeping track of any changes is to keep a log . Write down the distance you walked and your pace, and alongside it, write down how you felt physically and mentally. Plotting any new or unusual aches or pains in diary form will help you to track the cause, and hopefully help you prevent them from reoccurring.

Your support team

Seek out and identify people who can assist you in keeping your body strong and healthy. In my support team, I have my doctor, a chiropractor, a podiatrist, and an acupuncturist. It is sensible to do your research in advance so that you know who to turn to if you do have an injury (*see pp188–189*).

I would also advise that you visit health specialists for maintenance sessions, not just when you experience pain. Lower back pain is common in power walking, and is usually due to a poor walking posture. Often people lean forward from the waist with rounded shoulders. The solution is to change your technique, but a visit to the chiropractor on a regular basis acts as a good injury-prevention measure.

Body-scanning

You can use a body-scan meditation to improve your awareness of your body. It teaches you the skill of moving through your body and becoming sensitive to any physical changes.
• Sit comfortably and shake out any tension in your limbs and torso. Take some deep breaths.
• Begin by focusing on the area at the top of your head, then move down over the scalp and forehead, noting any tightness or pressure.
• Move your attention to your face. This is a common area of tension, so check that your eyes are soft and your mouth, tongue, and jaw are relaxed.

• Continue moving down your neck, into your throat, and then into the shoulders, arms, and hands. Again, note any subtle sensations.

• Feel the movement in your ribs and diaphragm with each inhalation and exhalation.

• As you focus on your belly and your lower back, notice your posture and any discomfort.

• Place your awareness on your hips, legs, and feet. Feel your feet firmly planted on the ground. Throughout the scan, breathe normally. If you find an area of tension, keep your awareness there until you feel the knots dissolve away. You may like to repeat the head-to-toe check one or more times, each time going deeper into relaxation.

Checklist for body wellness

Walking is a low-impact sport, so injuries are few and most are preventable, provided you listen to your body and adhere to some simple rules:

Footwear Wear the correct shoes and socks, and possibly orthotics to prevent injury to many parts of the body (see pp18–23).

Warm up and cool down Lengthened and warm muscles are less likely to be injured during a walk. Bringing the muscles slowly back into their resting state after exercise is essential (see pp68–72).

Stretching and strengthening Stretch every day to be sure your muscles have a full range of motion, and definitely stretch after every walk (see pp60–72). Follow a strengthening regimen on a daily basis if possible so that your muscles can cope with your training program (see pp52–59).

Rest days Without rest, your body will become worn down and unable to repair itself after an intense workout. If you walk fast or for a long distance one day, go slowly or for a shorter walk the next.

Overtraining Being overambitious can have a negative effect on your training. Work within your limits and build up your speed and distances slowly, particularly after an injury.

Cross-training When your body is tired from walking, try going for a swim or cycle ride instead, so that you use different muscles (see pp134–139).

Change your surface Depending on your injury, it could be that pounding on a hard surface is exacerbating it, so walk slowly on grass or a treadmill for a softer workout (see pp112–113).

Take care of your feet Rough skin causes blisters, and these can ruin, or even stop, a walk (see pp122–125).

PEDICURE

A monthly pedicure will give you pretty feet, and help to prevent blisters and bruised toes. Even if you can only spare 20 minutes, make your pedicure as luxurious and as special as you can. To finish, you may like to buff your nails to a natural shine. Add a dot of cocoa butter to each nail, then buff with a soft cloth or a ready-made nail buffer.

> **YOU WILL NEED**
> A bowl of warm water • nail clippers • nail file • pumice stone • body moisturizer or foot cream • essential oils • cuticle cream • cuticle stick • warm towels • thin cotton socks

1 Remove rough or hard skin from the foot. This is usually easier to do when the feet are dry. Rough skin tends to form on the heel, ball of the foot, and side of the big toe. When left to build up, it can cause blisters by rubbing on your shoes or socks when you are walking. Use a pumice stone, a callus reducer, or a good foot scrub to rub away hard skin gently, but don't overdo it.

2 Once you have removed any dry skin, soak your feet in a bowl of warm water for 5 minutes or so. Add 2–3 drops of essential oils, such as tea tree (antiseptic), or peppermint (energizing). Lavender essential oil is good for relaxation and balancing, and is one of my favorites.

4 Gently massage cuticle cream into the base of each nail and then push back each cuticle with a cuticle stick. It is better not to cut cuticles, since this actually encourages more growth.

3 Carefully dry your feet, paying special attention between your toes. Clip your toenails straight across, then use a nail file to smooth along the edge of each nail, stroking lightly in one direction. Make sure that corners are smooth and that there are no sharp edges. It helps to keep your nails short for power walking. If your nails are long, they can hit the toe box of your shoe as you push off, which can lead to bruised toes and black nails (*see p130*).

5 At this point you might like to give yourself a foot massage (*see p124*), but if you are short on time, smooth a nourishing body cream or oil into your feet. Put on cotton socks afterward to allow the moisturizer to soak in.

MASSAGE YOUR FEET

Massaging your feet is a powerful way to ease tension and relax your whole body. There is no time limit, but a minimum of 5–6 repetitions of each movement is much more relaxing than moving on to the next step too quickly. You will need essential oils, a base oil such as almond oil, and two towels.

BE AWARE Always check with a qualified aromatherapist before using any essential oils during pregnancy or if you have a medical condition. Use almond oil on its own if you are unsure.

1 Make up a massage oil consisting of 3 drops to 2 tsp (10ml) base oil. A combination of lavender, marjoram, and neroli makes a very relaxing mix. Prepare your hands by putting a few drops of oil into your palms and massaging your hands together until they feel soft and warm. Hold your foot sandwiched between your hands for a few moments, then stroke your foot with gentle sweeps toward your body, one hand behind the other.

2 Massage each toe using your thumbs. Continue by gliding your thumbs along the top of your foot toward your ankle and then back toward your toes, fanning your thumbs out to the side as you glide.

3 Start to loosen your toes by sandwiching them between your palms and rotating them clockwise and then counterclockwise.

4 Massage each toe again, this time with your thumb and forefinger, giving them a light squeeze and a roll. Finally, gently pull each toe in turn toward you.

5 Using gliding movements, run your thumbs between the four tendons on the top of your foot, moving toward the ankle.

7 Massage around the ankle and Achilles tendon area, making small, firm rotations. This feels instantly relaxing because we hold a great deal of tension in our ankles. Complete the massage by stroking the foot. Wrap it in a warm towel or blanket while you work on the other foot.

6 Firmly massage the sole of your foot. Use your thumbs to ease out from the center to the outer edges. Find a good reflexology book to tell you more about the powerful effect that massaging points on the feet has on the rest of your body.

STAYING INJURY-FREE

By strengthening the parts of the body most used in power walking—notably the knees, shins, ankles, and hips—you can help to prevent injuries. If you suffer an injury, return to training only after you are fully healed. Even then, the damaged area will be weakened and susceptible to further problems, so when you begin walking again, take it at a slower pace.

Shin splints

Causes and symptoms The calf muscles and the muscles on the front of the shin are probably used more in power walking than in any other sport. The technique (*see pp42–43*) is a distinct way of walking that puts pressure on these muscles to work hard. As a result of this, beginners and over-ambitious experienced walkers can feel a burning, throbbing, or aching sensation, or in milder cases just tenderness, on the front of the shin. Excessive pronation (*see pp18–19*) can also be a cause.

Usually the walker will have been training faster, or for a longer distance, than his or her fitness and ability allow. The muscles are being asked to work in a way they are not used to. A sign of shin splints is that the pain will subside while walking, but will return when you stop.

Treatment and prevention Wrap a bag of frozen peas in a towel and place the ice pack on the shin for around 15 minutes, three times a day, to relieve the muscle ache and inflammation. To relieve the pain and inflammation you can also use a mentholated ointment such as Tiger Balm, an Epsom salt bath,

CAUTION Any health conditions that you feel may be aggravated through power walking should be discussed with your doctor before you begin. Never ignore serious pain or leave any condition or injury untreated as you may cause irreparable damage. The information on these pages is a guide only. If in any doubt, contact your doctor.

or an anti-inflammatory. Rest from power walking until you feel comfortable again. When you begin walking, go back a few stages in your training and build up the speed and distance you walk more slowly.

To prevent this injury from recurring, or from appearing to begin with, you need to increase the strength and flexibility in your calf and shin muscles. This can be achieved through regular stretching (*see opposite and p129*). Start stretching the shins and calves gently every day. Also, look into the fit of your shoes, and make sure they are not too big or too tight, causing your toes to grip.

Sprains and strains

Causes and symptoms A sprain is an injury to a ligament that supports a joint, and usually occurs as a result of a fall or a twist. This type of injury can range from first-degree, which is a stretching of the ligament, to third-degree, the complete separation of the ligament from the bone or even a broken bone. Sprains can take weeks or months to heal.

A strain is an injury to muscles and tendons. These usually come about because of muscle overuse and can range from a minute tear in the muscle to a complete separation of the muscle-tendon-bone attachment.

Both injuries will usually result in painful swelling, inflammation, cramping, and weakness. Sometimes you may be aware of the strain at the time it takes place, or you may notice the pain when you have finished your walk.

QUAD AND ANKLE STRETCH

This exercise will help prevent shin splints and sprains and strains (*see opposite*), and plantar fasciitis (*see p130*). Your quads will receive a good stretch and your ankles will be stretched and strengthened as you lift onto your toe. The lift will also strengthen the calves and provide a stretch down the front of the shin.

1 Stand tall in a good posture. If you need to, place one hand on a wall for support. Bend your right leg and, holding your right ankle with your right hand, pull your foot toward your bottom. Keep your knees together and hips square to the front. Tense your buttock muscles to intensify the stretch.

2 Rise up onto the ball of your left foot and hold the position for 4 seconds. Then slowly bring the foot back down to the floor. Repeat the sequence 10 times and then repeat on the opposite leg.

Treatment and prevention The treatment for either of these injuries is to apply the RICE rule: rest, ice, compression, and elevation. Apply an ice pack to the area for 15 minutes, three times a day. Use a wide elastic bandage to wrap up and compress the area, tight enough that you feel some pain relief, but not so tight that the blood supply is cut off. To relieve the pain and inflammation you can also try a mentholated ointment such as Tiger Balm, an Epsom salt bath, or an anti-inflammatory.

Seek professional advice for both conditions because they are painful, they can be serious, and it can be difficult for you to ascertain the degree of injury without a proper examination.

Once the swelling has subsided and the injury is healing, gently begin stretching and strengthening the area (*see p127, p129, p131, and pp52–73*). It is important to keep the area mobile and flexible so that the joints and muscles can heal back to their original strength.When you begin walking, go back a few stages in your training schedule and build up the speed and distance you walk more slowly.

Blisters

Causes and symptoms Blisters are caused by continual rubbing against the skin. A bubble of fluid forms, pocketed between the top layers of skin, and when pressure is applied it feels painful.

Poorly fitting shoes are a common cause of blisters. Socks that are too big, too small, or too old and worn can also result in blisters. Other causes are rough skin or wet feet, either from extreme sweating or walking in rain.

Treatment and prevention The standard advice is to let the fluid subside naturally, and if this hasn't happened after 24 hours, to lance the bubble to drain the fluid. I find blisters don't heal quickly unless you lance the bubble immediately. You can sterilize the needle with a liquid antiseptic, in boiling water, or by heating it in a flame. Pierce two little holes, at either end of the blister. Using sterile gauze, press down gently to remove the liquid.

Wipe the area with an antiseptic solution, and then cover with nonallergenic dressing tape, not cotton. This will form a replacement for the skin, allowing the blister to heal in half the time.

If blisters continually return in the same place, make sure that you have the correct shoes for walking and that they fit properly (*see pp18– 23*). If you suspect your socks are the problem (*see p27*), try a different kind. Try covering your feet in petroleum jelly or talcum powder. These act as a barrier and protect the feet from being rubbed. Regular pedicures can also help (*see pp122–123*). Or try a "blister blocker." This is a soft resin that is worked into the skin using your fingers. Make sure you blend the edges so that the resin becomes almost a part of your foot.

Athlete's foot

Causes and symptoms This is a fungus that appears between the toes and on the soles of the feet as cracks of red, flaky, itchy skin that can be quite painful. It can cross-infect from foot to nail or nail to foot.

Treatment and prevention Apply an antifungal (fungicidal) cream to the infected areas as directed on the packaging. There are many products available. If athlete's foot returns, as it often does, treat it with a different brand of cream, since the fungus may form a tolerance to your usual brand. Continue treating the area for two weeks after the symptoms have disappeared because the fungus can still remain up to this point.

To help prevent a return of the fungus, keep your feet clean and dry at all times. Wear socks made of synthetic fabrics that will wick moisture away from your skin. It is important also to treat your shoes and socks, because washing them is not enough to destroy the fungus.

HEEL-TO-TOE ROCK

This movement helps to prevent shin splints and sprains and strains (*see p126*) by strengthening your shins, calves, and ankles. If you have a weakness in this area, or are a beginner to power walking, this is a very useful move for you to practice. Spend 5 minutes a day on this to enhance your technique.

1 Stand with feet a little less than shoulder-width apart, with your arms and hands hanging loosely by your sides. Legs are straight but knees are soft, and not locked. Bring your weight forward onto the balls of your feet, using your arms to balance you.

2 Using the momentum of your swing and your arms, rock back onto your heels. Keep your knees soft. Repeat the rocking motion 5 times forward and back, rest for 1 minute, then rock forward and back a further 5 times.

Black toenails

Causes and symptoms Black toenails are usually caused by shoes that are too small. Each time you push off from your toes as you walk, the toes bang against the end of the toe box in the shoe. Over time, this bruises the toes and causes a pooling of blood under the nail, which then blackens. The toe will be painful and will throb under the pressure of the blood that has collected.

Treatment and prevention It is possible to preserve your toenail by lancing it with a sterilized needle through the nail. This is painless, but must be done within an hour of the black toenail's first appearance. If you don't catch it early enough, or if it isn't too painful, leave it to heal naturally. Over the next few months the nail will fall off, and new nail will have grown underneath. Wear correctly fitting shoes to stop this from occurring, and try wearing thicker socks to cushion your toes.

Ingrown toenails

Causes and symptoms Ingrown nails occur mostly on the big toe and may be caused by poorly fitting shoes. How you cut and file your toenails may also encourage the toenail to grow into the skin, especially if the toenail is curved or has been cut too short on the sides of the nail. Ingrown nails can be very painful, particularly when the shoe adds pressure to the nail. The skin around the nail will be red and inflamed, and may become infected.

Treatment and prevention To reduce any swelling and discomfort, soak the affected foot in a bowl of warm water to which you have added 2–4 drops of tea tree essential oil or 1–2 tablespoons of salt at least once a day. If you are unable to cut the nail because it has become embedded in the skin, see a podiatrist, or your doctor.

Always cut toenails in a straight line to prevent the inward growth. Make sure you file any sharp corners with an emery board.

Plantar fasciitis

Causes and symptoms Plantar fasciitis is an inflammation of the plantar fascia, a band of thick tissue that binds the muscle in the sole of the foot, caused by too much stress being placed on the area. It is easy to detect because the pain in your heel will be felt immediately as you get up in the morning or after sitting for some time, and then lessens as the day goes on. The pain is often described as feeling like a "bone bruise."

Common causes are continuous standing, being overweight, having flat feet (especially if they overpronate, *see p18*) or high-arched feet, worn-out shoes that allow overpronation, or a tightness in the Achilles tendon.

Treatment and prevention Rest until the pain disappears. Apply an ice pack to the area for 15–20 minutes four times a day and elevate the foot whenever possible. Healing cannot be rushed, so you may have to be patient.

If you still feel pain after prolonged treatment, visit a podiatrist. You may need heel cups and padding or orthotics (*see p20*) to treat the real problem instead of the symptoms. Roll a small ball underneath your foot, pressing down to get the depth of massage you require. Work on stretching and strengthening the Achilles tendon and calf muscles (*see p129*). Check that your shoes are not too worn and support your arches (*see pp18–23*).

Swollen fingers

Causes and symptoms Fingers swell and become cold when the blood supply is depleted. This can be caused by having your arms and hands down at your sides while walking.

Treatment and prevention Keep your arms at a 90-degree angle (*see p44*) and regularly clench and unclench your fists. By using the correct arm movement, you encourage good blood flow. Wearing gloves also makes a big difference.

BALL SQUATS

This exercise is excellent for preventing strains and sprains (*see p127*). It improves strength and tones up your thighs, hamstrings, buttocks, and quads. Using the ball helps you to put extra weight into your heels, which increases the intensity of the squat. Controlling the ball also gives your lower back a workout.

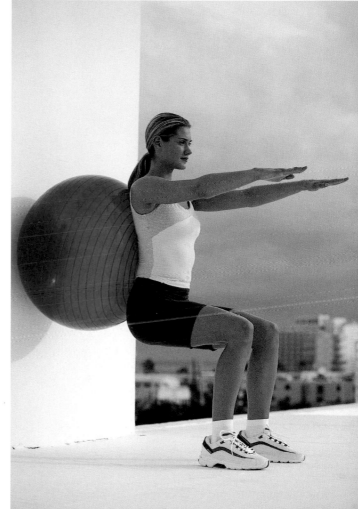

1 Place the exercise ball between you and the wall. It should rest behind your lower and middle back. Your knees should be hip-width apart and only slightly bent. Stretch your arms out in front of you to help you balance.

2 Slide slowly down the wall, rolling the ball against it. Stop when you reach a sitting position with knees bent at a 90-degree angle. Keep your back straight. Hold for 4 counts, then slowly return to the start position. Repeat 5 times, then rest. The slower you do this, the more intense the squat. Increase the number of counts as you grow stronger.

TRAINING PROGRAMS

Making a commitment to a training program can feel a little overwhelming, but I hope you will feel excited, too. The rewards and satisfaction of sticking to an exercise regime come not just from reaching a goal, but from discovering new strengths and abilities within yourself, and relishing the achievements that you have gained along the way.

"In each of us are places where we have never gone. Only by pressing the limits do you ever find them."

DR JOYCE BROTHERS

CROSS-TRAINING

There is a saying that "a change is as good as a rest," and this is certainly true for the body. Power walking works your calves, hamstrings, and glutes particularly hard, so to balance this, you need to do activities that work other muscles, or that challenge the same muscles in a different way. Days when you cross-train allow your key walking muscles to recover and actually grow stronger.

Any form of exercise is suitable for your cross-training, including swimming, cycling, dancing, rollerblading, orienteering, and working out in a gym. Don't feel restricted to this list, though. Any exercise carried out for 30 minutes that raises your heart rate will be beneficial to you.

Swimming

The focus in swimming is on the upper body and torso, and it is therefore excellent cross-training for walking. It can give you a good overall cardiovascular workout, though it is not as easy to increase your heart rate as when you are walking. Try building up to 30 minutes of continuous swimming, or try interval training (*see p111*) in the pool.

You might also like to try water aerobics or pool-walking or -running, which involves walking or running lengths of the pool. This really tones muscle because of the resistance the water creates against your body, making it an excellent way to burn calories.

Cycling

Walking uses the hamstrings and glutes, while riding a bike is good for working the quadriceps, which makes it another excellent cross-training exercise to do with walking. Cycling will keep you aerobically fit, increase your levels of strength and stamina, and support your muscle function. It is a nonimpact sport that specifically works the abductors, which are important for balance and coordination.

There are many types of bikes available, including those suitable for speed and touring, mountain bikes for off-road trails and orienteering, and racing bikes and tandems. Contact a specialist if you are considering buying a bike to make sure you buy the right one for you. Research different clubs and organizations to discover what type of cycling activity appeals to you.

To benefit fully from the endurance and strength you can gain from cycling, you need to be able to cycle for 30 minutes at a sustained speed. It is advisable to work at strengthening your knees, especially if you are going off-road.

Dancing

All types of dancing are suitable for fitness, including salsa, jazz, belly, swing, hip-hop, tango, modern, and old-time. Any of these styles of dance will develop whole-body coordination because your body is required to move in every direction. Dancing is social, great fun, and a healthy way to get fit.

Depending on the type of dancing and how vigorous you are, it can give you a cardiovascular workout and will certainly put your core stability muscles to the test. Salsa, for example, is excellent for working your abdominal obliques.

Again, depending on your choice of dance, it can be weight-bearing and consequently will help to either strengthen bones or maintain bone density and prevent osteoporosis. Vigorous, sustained dancing for an hour burns approximately 300 calories, which is the same amount as walking or cycling. As with most forms of exercise, to get the maximum benefit, you should aim to dance for 30 minutes continuously. As with any vigorous exercise, you should warm up and do some stretches before starting. Cool down and stretch at the end.

Rollerblading

For an activity that can look so effortless, rollerblading burns up a surprisingly large amount of energy, especially when you are learning. It is tremendous for developing core stability and coordination, and it particularly works the muscles of the legs and buttocks. Because a lot of your control and power comes from the lower body and knees, work at strengthening these muscles with lunges (*see p137*) and ball squats (*see p131*).

Orienteering

If you like the excitement of exploring and enjoy being in the countryside, then this is the sport for you (*see p103*). The routes with their control points are usually through forests and rugged terrains, and vary in lengths from 1 mile (2km) for children to 7 miles (12km) for experienced adult orienteers. You can make the workout as hard or easy as you want by running, jogging, or walking. It will test your endurance and give you a whole-body workout.

Kettlebells

Kettlebells come in a variety of weights and look like a cannonball with a handle. The beauty of this workout is that it can be tailored to suit all ages and fitness abilities. Being both a cardio and strengthening workout, it also comes with a long

Regular kettlebell workouts can help to keep you lean and strong, improve posture, aid weight control, and develop good coordination and mental focus.

list of all-around benefits. These include improving muscle tone, core strength, flexibility, and balance, as well as developing good posture.

This is an easy workout to do at home, ideally 2–3 times a week, but even 5 minutes a day can reap benefits. It uses just four basic movements in endless variation. To get started, there are a number of good websites that you can join to receive technique advice and workouts (*see pp188–189*).

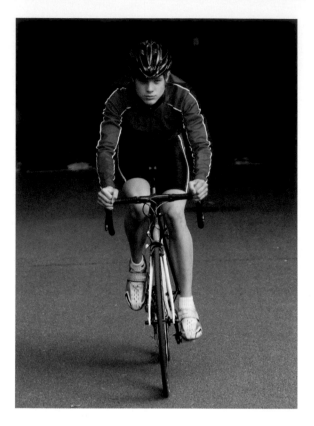

In the gym

Working out in a gym can be a great addition to your fitness program, particularly on dark winter nights, in bad weather, or if you are recovering from an injury. Most gyms offer a good range of cross-training classes, from kick-boxing to Pilates. The variety will help to keep you motivated on your fitness plan. One of the advantages of using equipment such as treadmills and weight machines in a gym is that they are often placed in front of mirrors so that you can continually check and correct your posture. In addition, you have experienced instructors on hand to give advice on using the equipment properly and safely. Use them to pick up exercises that you could do at home and include them in your daily stretch and strengthen routine (*see p73*). I have included here a selection of exercises that can be done at home or in a gym.

Cycling outdoors is a good sport for reducing stress because most people find it a pleasurable form of exercise, and it is an activity suitable for all ages.

The lunge opposite works on strengthening your lower body, and is followed by two excellent exercises for building the muscles in the arms.

Walking on a treadmill

If you are new to using a treadmill, you will find that the display panel offers quite a few readings and programs to master, such as a calorie counter, heart-rate monitor, speedometer, pace function, and hill walking and terrain programs. They are easy to use, and your gym instructor will be able to answer any questions.

The sensation of walking on a treadmill is very different from walking on a road, and can feel quite bouncy. This makes walking, jogging, or running easier and faster and puts less strain on your joints. However, a common mistake people make is to walk with the treadmill in a flat position. Although your body is moving forward with each stride, the treadmill does not require the same level of exertion and muscle power from you as the road does because of the soft surface. In fact, walking flat on a treadmill will eventually lead to weakened muscles. Always set the treadmill to an incline of at least 1 percent, even as a beginner, to be sure you are replicating your road-walking speed.

Use the heart-rate monitor function to make sure that you match your pace and exertion to that of your road walking. The procedure for stretching, warming up, and cooling down is the same as usual (*see pp68–72*), except that you get off the machine to stretch. Do not walk barefoot on a treadmill— this can be dangerous.

Creating your own hills and terrain on a treadmill can be challenging and fun. The options allow you to build programs of varying lengths, inclines, and intensity. Moderate-to-steep inclines will give you a good workout, make you a stronger walker, and still offer a low risk of injury. However, inclines of 15 percent or more will place stress on your shins and ankles and so should not be attempted too often.

Overtraining

Sometimes trying to fit in a walking program when you have other stresses in your life can lead to overtraining syndrome and burnout. Even if you are not suffering from stress, if you work too hard at your training, and do not take essential rest periods (see pp120–121), you may overtrain.

The symptoms of overtraining manifest themselves in different ways in different people, but typically include fatigue, altered sleep patterns, loss of appetite, unquenchable thirst, muscle aches even after a light workout, being depressed or anxious, feeling impatient or easily upset, and having a high resting heart rate. However, you should check that there is no underlying illness that is responsible for the above symptoms.

If you feel you have overtrained, take immediate steps by cutting down on your training. Start keeping a log to monitor your progress, and include details of how you feel both physically and emotionally. Record your sleeping patterns and how restful they are. Treat yourself to a massage or a week's rest. It is easier to prevent overtraining than to recover from it.

LUNGES

These strengthen and tone your quads, hamstrings, calves, and glutes. The abductors and adductors are also used to stabilize you. To increase the challenge, do lunges in bare feet. Weights are optional, but using them will bring faster results. Keep your movements slow and controlled for maximum benefit. Complete 2 sets of 5 lunges on each leg.

1 Check your posture and tighten your abdominals. Take one full stride back with your left foot and land on your toes. Feel equally balanced on both feet.

2 With your back straight and shoulders relaxed, lunge down to a count of four, bending both knees until they are at 90 degrees. The right knee should not extend over your toes. Hold for 4 counts, then rise to 4 counts.

BICEP CURLS

These curls focus on strengthening and toning the biceps. Doing this exercise regularly will give you great definition in the front of your arms. By doing the curls with one foot on an exercise ball, you are required to use your balance. At the top of the movement, concentrate on flexing your biceps.

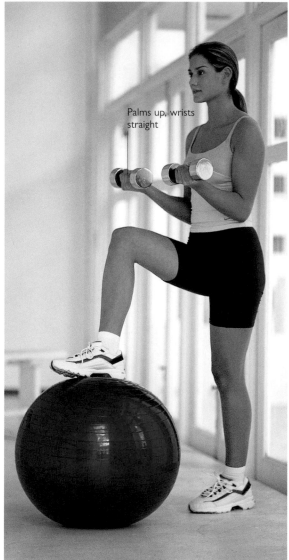

Palms up, wrists straight

1 Take one weight in each hand and place your right foot flat on the ball. Focus and stabilize yourself before starting the curls. Check your posture and keep your eyes looking directly ahead. Be aware of your core stability and balance.

2 Hold the weights at right angles to your body. Slowly lift the weights to the count of 4. Hold for 4 counts, then slowly come down to a count of 4. Complete 2 sets of 5 curls, then change legs and repeat.

TRICEP DIPS

Here you use your own body weight as resistance instead of free weights. This exercise is great for toning and strengthening the triceps in the back of your arms.

If possible, do tricep dips in the same session as the bicep curls so that both sides of the arms are worked together.

1 Sit on the front edge of a bench or chair. Place your hands by your sides with fingers facing forward. Lift your weight up onto your arms. Straighten your arms but don't lock your elbows. Keep your knees at 90 degrees and your heels slightly forward from your knees.

2 Lower yourself toward the floor, elbows pointing backward, until your arms are bent at 90 degrees. Hold the position for a second, then push yourself up slowly through your arms as you exhale deeply. Repeat 10–15 times.

BEGINNER: STAGE 1

This program is designed for anyone who is starting a fitness regime for the very first time, or for people who have not been active for a long period and feel as though they are starting from scratch. The goal is to reach a short-distance walking speed of 1 mile (1.6km) in 15–18 minutes.

Week 1

Walk ½–1 mile (0.8–1.6km) and decide which distance is the best starting point for you. A steady pace means you do not need to push yourself hard, and can concentrate on achieving the distance. You may already have more stamina than you think if you are active in your daily life. It is more important to get used to the routine of getting exercise than to worry about speed, but no matter how slow you walk, try to keep a steady and continuous pace. Stretch for around 5–10 minutes on your rest days to improve your flexibility and strength.

Week 2

Introduce stretching into your walk days as well as your rest days by warming up and cooling down. To warm up, stretch for 5 minutes after the first 10 minutes of your walk. To cool down, slow your pace about 10 minutes from the end of your walk and stretch immediately after. Start to work on your technique and get used to using your body.

Week 4

Start to introduce other activities into your schedule in week 4. It can be anything you enjoy, such as swimming or weight-training.

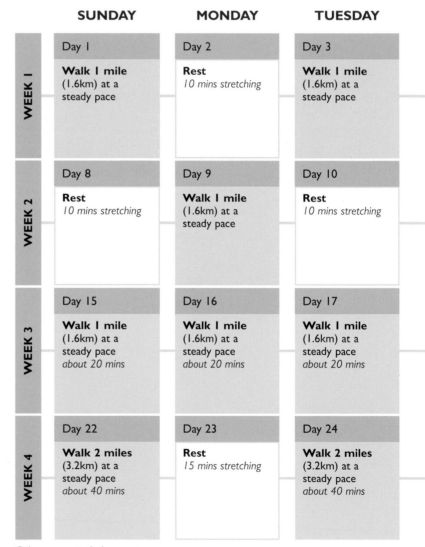

	SUNDAY	MONDAY	TUESDAY
WEEK 1	Day 1 — **Walk 1 mile** (1.6km) at a steady pace	Day 2 — **Rest** *10 mins stretching*	Day 3 — **Walk 1 mile** (1.6km) at a steady pace
WEEK 2	Day 8 — **Rest** *10 mins stretching*	Day 9 — **Walk 1 mile** (1.6km) at a steady pace	Day 10 — **Rest** *10 mins stretching*
WEEK 3	Day 15 — **Walk 1 mile** (1.6km) at a steady pace *about 20 mins*	Day 16 — **Walk 1 mile** (1.6km) at a steady pace *about 20 mins*	Day 17 — **Walk 1 mile** (1.6km) at a steady pace *about 20 mins*
WEEK 4	Day 22 — **Walk 2 miles** (3.2km) at a steady pace *about 40 mins*	Day 23 — **Rest** *15 mins stretching*	Day 24 — **Walk 2 miles** (3.2km) at a steady pace *about 40 mins*

Other pages to help you
• Any other activity, see pp134–137 • Interval training, see pp110–111

When starting to power walk, it is important to develop stamina and strength before you deal with speed. Therefore, weeks 1–6 focus on developing strength, flexibility, and stamina. You will find that as you work on these, you will naturally speed up. In weeks 7–12, you will start to develop speed. Ease yourself slowly into exercise, especially if you are unfit. Use the times given here as approximate goals for which you should aim. It is important to commit yourself to daily activity, so only miss a maximum of one walk a week and never miss a stretching session.

Key

	Walk days
	Other activity days
	Rest days

WEDNESDAY	THURSDAY	FRIDAY	SATURDAY	
Day 4	Day 5	Day 6	Day 7	Total
Rest *10 mins stretching*	**Walk 1 mile (1.6km) at a steady pace**	**Rest** *10 mins stretching*	**Walk 1 mile (1.6km) at a steady pace**	**4 miles (6.4km)**
Day 11	Day 12	Day 13	Day 14	Total
Walk 1 mile (1.6km) at a steady pace	**Rest** *10 mins stretching*	**Walk 1 mile (1.6km) at a steady pace**	**Rest** *10 mins stretching*	**3 miles (4.8km)**
Day 18	Day 19	Day 20	Day 21	Total
Rest *10 mins stretching*	**Walk 1 mile (1.6km) at a steady pace** *about 20 mins*	**Walk 1 mile (1.6km) at a steady pace** *about 20 mins*	**Walk 1 mile (1.6km) at a steady pace** *about 20 mins*	**6 miles (9.6km)**
Day 25	Day 26	Day 27	Day 28	Total
Walk 2 miles (3.2km) at a steady pace *about 40 mins*	**Rest** *10 mins stretching*	**Any other activity** *for a minimum of 15 mins*	**Rest** *10 mins stretching*	**6 miles (9.6km)**

Exercise pages
• Stretching exercises, see pp60–67 • Warming up and cooling down, see Warm-up and cooldown plan p72 • Exercise-ball training, see pp56–59, p131, p139

BEGINNER: STAGE 2

Weeks 5–6

You are walking farther and more often, so stretching is vital. From week 5 on, you should spend 15–20 seconds on each stretch. Start to work on taking different routes to introduce variety and interest to your walks.

Weeks 7–8

As you begin moving at a faster pace, you are working on strength and developing technique. At a faster pace, you are walking with purpose and should feel that you are exerting yourself; however, you should still be able to talk as you walk. If you do not feel ready for this, go back to week 5 and complete the last 2 weeks again. If you feel fine and ready to move on, then continue into weeks 7 and 8.

Try tracking 10,000 steps and begin to include it into your day's walking. It is not important to reach that total, but quite often it becomes a personal challenge to see the steps racking up. The more you walk, the faster and farther you will be able to walk.

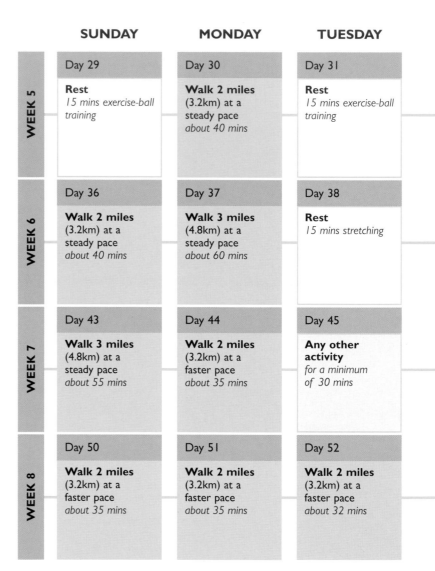

	SUNDAY	MONDAY	TUESDAY
WEEK 5	Day 29 **Rest** *15 mins exercise-ball training*	Day 30 **Walk 2 miles** (3.2km) at a steady pace *about 40 mins*	Day 31 **Rest** *15 mins exercise-ball training*
WEEK 6	Day 36 **Walk 2 miles** (3.2km) at a steady pace *about 40 mins*	Day 37 **Walk 3 miles** (4.8km) at a steady pace *about 60 mins*	Day 38 **Rest** *15 mins stretching*
WEEK 7	Day 43 **Walk 3 miles** (4.8km) at a steady pace *about 55 mins*	Day 44 **Walk 2 miles** (3.2km) at a faster pace *about 35 mins*	Day 45 **Any other activity** *for a minimum of 30 mins*
WEEK 8	Day 50 **Walk 2 miles** (3.2km) at a faster pace *about 35 mins*	Day 51 **Walk 2 miles** (3.2km) at a faster pace *about 35 mins*	Day 52 **Walk 2 miles** (3.2km) at a faster pace *about 32 mins*

Other pages that will help you
• Any other activity, see pp134–137 • Interval training, see pp110–111

WEDNESDAY	THURSDAY	FRIDAY	SATURDAY	
Day 32	**Day 33**	**Day 34**	**Day 35**	**Total**
Any other activity *for a minimum of 30 mins*	**Walk 3 miles** (4.8km) at a steady pace *about 60 mins*	**Rest** *15 mins exercise-ball training*	**Walk 2 miles** (3.2km) at a steady pace *about 40 mins*	**7 miles** (11.2km)
Day 39	**Day 40**	**Day 41**	**Day 42**	**Total**
Any other activity *for a minimum of 30 mins*	**Walk 2 miles** (3.2km) at a steady pace *about 40 mins*	**Walk 2 miles** (3.2km) at a steady pace *about 40 mins*	**Walk 2 miles** (3.2km) at a steady pace *about 40 mins*	**11 miles** (17.6km)
Day 46	**Day 47**	**Day 48**	**Day 49**	**Total**
Rest *15 mins stretching*	**Walk 3 miles** (4.8km) at a steady pace *about 55 mins*	**Walk 2 miles** (3.2km) at a faster pace *about 35 mins*	**Walk 1 mile** (1.6km) at top speed *about 18 mins*	**11 miles** (17.6km)
Day 53	**Day 54**	**Day 55**	**Day 56**	**Total**
Walk 3 miles (4.8km) at a steady pace *about 50 mins*	**Any other activity** *for a minimum of 15 mins*	**Rest** *15 mins stretching*	**Walk 2 miles** (3.2km) at a faster pace *about 32 mins*	**11 miles** (17.6km)

Key

Walk days

Other activity days

Rest days

Exercise pages
• Stretching exercises, see pp60–67 • Warming up and cooling down, see Warm-up and cooldown plan p72 • Exercise-ball training, see pp56–59, p131, p139

BEGINNER: STAGE 3

Weeks 9–12

Walking at speed means you need to work harder and push forward a little more. Listen to your body, and if you find the pace too hard, take it down a notch. If you wish, you can introduce interval training. This is when you walk as fast as you can for anything starting from 30 seconds to a minute, and then walk at a relaxed pace for double that time (so 1–2 minutes). You can repeat this as many times as you wish within one session, building up the times as you progress. Just be aware that it is an intense form of training, and you may very well feel it the next day.

By the end of week 12, you should feel confident in walking regularly and begin to feel fitter and more toned.

When you have completed this program, you may wish to try the intermediate program (pp146–151) or, depending on your ultimate goal, the short-distance program (pp158–163).

	SUNDAY	MONDAY	TUESDAY
WEEK 9	Day 57 **Walk 2 miles** (3.2km) at a faster pace *about 30–34 mins*	Day 58 **Walk 3 miles** (4.8km) at a steady pace *about 51 mins*	Day 59 **Any other activity** *for a minimum of 30 mins*
WEEK 10	Day 64 **Walk 3 miles** (4.8km) at a faster pace *about 50 mins*	Day 65 **Walk 3 miles** (4.8km) at a faster pace *about 50 mins*	Day 66 **Rest** *15 mins stretching*
WEEK 11	Day 71 **Walk 3 miles** (4.8km) at a faster pace *about 45–50 mins*	Day 72 **Walk 3 miles** (4.8km) at a faster pace *about 45–50 mins*	Day 73 **Rest** *15 mins stretching*
WEEK 12	Day 78 **Walk 4 miles** (6.4km) at a steady pace *about 68 mins*	Day 79 **Walk 3 miles** (4.8km) at a top speed *about 45 mins*	Day 80 **Any other activity** *for a minimum of 30 mins*

Other pages that will help you
• Any other activity, see pp134–137 • Interval training, see pp110–111

WEDNESDAY	THURSDAY	FRIDAY	SATURDAY	
Day 60 **Walk 2 miles** **(3.2km) at a** **faster pace** *about 30–34 mins*	**Day 61** **Walk 3 miles** **(4.8km) at a** **faster pace** *about 48 mins*	**Day 62** **Rest** *15 mins exercise-ball training*	**Day 63** **Walk 2 miles** **(3.2km) at a** **faster pace** *about 30–34 mins*	**Total** **12 miles** **(19.2km)**
Day 67 **Any other activity** *for a minimum of 30 mins*	**Day 68** **Walk 2 miles** **(3.2km)** *about 30 mins*	**Day 69** **Walk 3 miles** **(4.8km) at a** **faster pace** *about 50 mins*	**Day 70** **Walk 3 miles** **(4.8km) at a** **faster pace** *about 50 mins*	**Total** **14 miles** **(22.4km)**
Day 74 **Any other activity** *for a minimum of 30 mins*	**Day 75** **Walk 3 miles** **(4.8km) at a** **faster pace** *about 45–50 mins*	**Day 76** **Walk 3 miles** **(4.8km) at a** **faster pace** *about 45–50 mins*	**Day 77** **Walk 3 miles** **(4.8km) at a** **faster pace** *about 45–50 mins*	**Total** **15 miles** **(24km)**
Day 81 **Walk 4 miles** **(6.4km) at a** **steady pace** *about 70–98 mins*	**Day 82** **Walk 3 miles** **(4.8km) at a** **top speed** *about 45–50 mins*	**Day 83** **Rest** *15 mins stretching*	**Day 84** **Walk 4 miles** **(6.4km) at a** **top speed** *about 60 mins*	**Total** **18 miles** **(28.8km)**

Key

- Walk days
- Other activity days
- Rest days

Exercise pages
- Stretching exercises, see pp60–67 • Warming up and cooling down, see Warm-up and cooldown plan p72 • Exercise-ball training, see pp56–59, p131, p139

INTERMEDIATE: STAGE 1

If you are able to walk 4 miles (6.4km) at a constant pace and want to take the next step in training, then you are ready for the intermediate program. Exercising and stretching on a daily basis will keep you fit, strengthen your body, make you leaner and more toned, and develop your speed and walking technique.

Weeks 1–2

The aim of this plan is to focus on developing core strength and stamina by not only walking longer distances at speed, but also combining it with other activities, including regular stretching. By including stretching in the warm-up and cooldown part of your walk, and also as part of your daily routine, you can alleviate tight muscles in your ankles, shins, and hips, which is very common when starting to walk fast over longer distances.

As for other activities, try either something that you know you will enjoy or something new that you have not tried before. By including sports such as swimming, cycling or dancing, it is a good way to cross-train and also add variety to your training week.

Weeks 3–4

Hill walking is introduced in week 3. You will either need to find a route that includes hills or resort to a treadmill. If you do the latter, always use it at a minimum setting of 2. The benefit of hill walking is that it is an excellent way to increase your walking strength.

Core stability sessions are also included in week 4. You can try Pilates, use an exercise ball, or swing a kettlebell. All really good core workouts that you can do at home or in a gym.

	SUNDAY	MONDAY	TUESDAY
WEEK 1	**Day 1** **Walk 3 miles (4.8km)** *about 45–55 mins + 15 mins stretch and strengthen*	**Day 2** **Any other activity** *for 30 mins*	**Day 3** **Rest** *15 mins stretch and strengthen*
WEEK 2	**Day 8** **Walk 4 miles (6.4km)** *about 60–68 mins + 15 mins stretch and strengthen*	**Day 9** **Rest** *15 mins stretch and strengthen*	**Day 10** **Walk 3 miles (4.8km)** *about 45–55 mins + 15 mins stretch and strengthen*
WEEK 3	**Day 15** **Rest** *15 mins stretch and strengthen*	**Day 16** **Walk 3 miles (4.8km)** *about 45–55 mins + 15 mins stretch and strengthen*	**Day 17** **Hill walking 3 miles (4.8km)** *about 50–55 mins + 15 mins stretch and strengthen*
WEEK 4	**Day 22** **Rest** *30 mins core stability training*	**Day 23** **Walk 6 miles (9.6km)** *about 90–100 mins + 15 mins stretch and strengthen*	**Day 24** **Rest** *15 mins stretch and strengthen*

Other pages to help you

• Using a heart-rate monitor, see pp32–35 • Any other activity, see pp134–137 • Hill walking, see pp112–113 • Using a pedometer, see pp36–37 • Interval training, see pp110–111 • Foods for fitness, see pp90–91 • Fit walking into your day, see pp94–95

To achieve results, you must be prepared to walk three to four times a week. Use this program as a guide to plan a training schedule that fits your life. Daily stretching and strengthening are important parts of the program and will make a big difference in your flexibility and strength, allowing you to progress more rapidly. It takes the body 4–6 weeks to get used to a new cardiovascular pattern, and it is better not to work on stamina and speed simultaneously. You will find that they eventually do come together during the course of the program. Use the times given here as approximate goals for which you should aim. Always follow a hard training day with an easier one.

Key

Walk days

Other activity days

Rest days

WEDNESDAY	THURSDAY	FRIDAY	SATURDAY	
Day 4	**Day 5**	**Day 6**	**Day 7**	**Total**
Walk 3 miles (4.8km) *about 45–55 mins + 15 mins stretch and strengthen*	**Rest** *15 mins stretch and strengthen*	**Walk 3 miles** (4.8km) *about 45–55 mins + 15 mins stretch and strengthen*	**Rest** *15 mins stretch and strengthen*	**9 miles** (14.4km)
Day 11	**Day 12**	**Day 13**	**Day 14**	**Total**
Rest *15 mins stretch and strengthen*	**Any other activity** *for a minimum of 15 mins*	**Rest** *15 mins stretch and strengthen*	**Walk 4 miles** (6.4km) *about 60–68 mins + 15 mins stretch and strengthen*	**11 miles** (17.6km)
Day 18	**Day 19**	**Day 20**	**Day 21**	**Total**
Rest *15 mins stretch and strengthen*	**Any other activity** *for a minimum of 30 mins*	**Walk 5 miles** (8km) *about 75–80 mins + 15 mins stretch and strengthen*	**Rest** *15 mins stretch and strengthen*	**11 miles** (17.6km)
Day 25	**Day 26**	**Day 27**	**Day 28**	**Total**
Walk 5 miles (8km) *about 75–80 mins + 15 mins stretch and strengthen*	**Rest** *15 mins stretch and strengthen*	**Walk 3 miles** (4.8km) *about 45–50 mins + 15 mins stretch and strengthen*	**Any other activity** *for a minimum of 30 mins*	**14 miles** (22.4km)

Exercise pages
- Warming up and cooling down, see Warm-up and cooldown plan p72 • Stretch and strengthen, see Stretching and strengthening plan p73
- Core stability training, see pp54–59

INTERMEDIATE: STAGE 2

Weeks 5–8

By week 5, you should be feeling stronger and have more energy. You will find that your speed will continue to develop over the next few weeks, particularly if you are also focusing on improving your technique.

Achieving a good heel strike and push-off while also keeping your arms at right angles and pumping them no higher than your shoulders can all feel like hard work, but it is worth persevering. It is almost impossible to increase your speed beyond 4–4½ miles an hour (6.5–7kph) without the use of good technique, particularly with the arms.

Wearing a fitness tracker or device is a great way of keeping a daily log. The more intense the challenge, the more that you will appreciate tracking your progress as stepping stones to your ultimate goal.

If you have not tried swinging a kettlebell yet, book a class to learn the basic movements.

	SUNDAY	MONDAY	TUESDAY
WEEK 5	Day 29 **Rest** *15 mins stretch and strengthen*	Day 30 **Walk 7 miles (11.2km)** *about 105–112 mins + 15 mins stretch and strengthen*	Day 31 **Rest** *15 mins stretch and strengthen*
WEEK 6	Day 36 **Walk 8 miles (12.9km)** *about 105–112 mins + 15 mins stretch and strengthen*	Day 37 **Rest** *15 mins stretch and strengthen*	Day 38 **Walk 6 miles (9.6km)** *about 90 mins + 15 mins stretch and strengthen*
WEEK 7	Day 43 **Walk 9 miles (14.4km)** *about 135–144 mins + 15 mins stretch and strengthen*	Day 44 **Rest** *15 mins stretch and strengthen*	Day 45 **Walk 5 miles (8km)** *about 75–80 mins + 15 mins stretch and strengthen*
WEEK 8	Day 50 **Rest** *15 mins stretch and strengthen*	Day 51 **Walk 5 miles (8km)** *about 75 mins + 15 mins stretch and strengthen*	Day 52 **Hill walking 3 miles (4.8km)** *about 50–55 mins + 15 mins stretch and strengthen*

Other pages to help you

• Using a heart-rate monitor, see pp32–35 • Any other activity, see pp134–137 • Hill walking, see pp112–113 • Using a pedometer, see pp36–37 • Interval training, see pp110–111
• Foods for fitness, see pp90–91 • Fit walking into your day, see pp94–95

WEDNESDAY	THURSDAY	FRIDAY	SATURDAY	
Day 32	**Day 33**	**Day 34**	**Day 35**	Total
Walk 6 miles (9.6km) *about 90–96 mins + 15 mins stretch and strengthen*	**Rest** *30 mins core stability training*	**Rest** *15 mins stretch and strengthen*	**Walk 4 miles** (6.4km) *about 60–64 mins + 15 mins stretch and strengthen*	**17 miles** (27.2km)
Day 39	**Day 40**	**Day 41**	**Day 42**	Total
Interval training 3 miles (4.8km) *about 45–50 mins + 15 mins stretch and strengthen*	**Rest** *15 mins stretch and strengthen*	**Any other activity** *for a minimum of 30 mins*	**Walk 4 miles** (6.4km) *about 60 mins + 15 mins stretch and strengthen*	**21 miles** (33.7km)
Day 46	**Day 47**	**Day 48**	**Day 49**	Total
Any other activity *for a minimum of 30 mins*	**Rest** *15 mins stretch and strengthen*	**Interval training 3 miles** (4.8km) *about 45–50 mins + 15 mins stretch and strengthen*	**Walk 7 miles** (11.2km) *about 105 mins + 15 mins stretch and strengthen*	**24 miles** (38.4km)
Day 53	**Day 54**	**Day 55**	**Day 56**	Total
Rest *15 mins stretch and strengthen*	**Walk 4 miles** (6.4km) *60–64 mins + 15 mins stretch and strengthen*	**Rest** *15 mins stretch and strengthen*	**Walk 9 miles** (14.4km) *135–144 mins + 15 mins stretch and strengthen*	**21 miles** (33.7km)

Key

Walk days

Other activity days

Rest days

Exercise pages
• Warming up and cooling down, see Warm-up and cooldown plan p72 • Stretch and strengthen, see Stretching and strengthening plan p73 • Exercise-ball training, see pp56–59, p131, p139

INTERMEDIATE: STAGE 3

Weeks 9–12

In these final weeks of the plan, you'll be reaching a level of fitness that will allow you to keep training and maintaining fitness at this regular pace. You can even consider joining a challenge if that is your goal.

Use your interval training as a way to increase the intensity of your workout and also your speed. However, it is advisable not to interval train on two consecutive days.

	SUNDAY	MONDAY	TUESDAY
WEEK 9	**Day 57** **Any other activity** *for a minimum of 30 mins*	**Day 58** **Rest** *15 mins stretch and strengthen*	**Day 59** **Interval training 3 miles** **(4.8km)** *about 45–50 mins + 15 mins stretch and strengthen*
WEEK 10	**Day 64** **Walk 10 miles** **(16km)** *about 150 mins + 15 mins stretch and strengthen*	**Day 65** **Rest** *15 mins stretch and strengthen*	**Day 66** **Interval training 4 miles** **(6.4km)** *about 58–60 mins + 15 mins stretch and strengthen*
WEEK 11	**Day 71** **Rest** *15 mins stretch and strengthen*	**Day 72** **Walk 5 miles** **(8km)** *about 75–80 mins + 15 mins stretch and strengthen*	**Day 73** **Rest** *15 mins stretch and strengthen*
WEEK 12	**Day 78** **Hill walking 4 miles** **(6.4km)** *about 60 mins + 15 mins stretch and strengthen*	**Day 79** **Rest** *15 mins stretch and strengthen*	**Day 80** **Walk 6 miles** **(9.6km)** *about 84–90 mins + 15 mins stretch and strengthen*

Other pages to help you
• Using a heart-rate monitor, see pp32–35 • Any other activity, see pp134–137 • Hill walking, see pp112–113 • Using a pedometer, see pp36–37 • Interval training, see pp110–111 • Foods for fitness, see pp90–91 • Fit walking into your day, see pp94–95

WEDNESDAY	THURSDAY	FRIDAY	SATURDAY	
Day 60	**Day 61**	**Day 62**	**Day 63**	**Total**
Rest *15 mins stretch and strengthen*	**Walk 5 miles (8km)** *about 70–75 mins + 15 mins stretch and strengthen*	**Walk 4 miles (6.4km)** *about 56–60 mins + 15 mins stretch and strengthen*	**Rest** *15 mins stretch and strengthen*	**12 miles (19.2km)**
Day 67	**Day 68**	**Day 69**	**Day 70**	**Total**
Walk 4 miles (6.4km) *about 60 mins + 15 mins stretch and strengthen*	**Rest** *15 mins stretch and strengthen*	**Any other activity** *for 60 mins*	**Walk 7 miles (11.2km)** *about 98 mins + 15 mins stretch and strengthen*	**25 miles (40km)**
Day 74	**Day 75**	**Day 76**	**Day 77**	**Total**
Interval training 4 miles (6.4km) *about 58–60 mins + 15 mins stretch and strengthen*	**Rest** *15 mins stretch and strengthen*	**Any other activity** *for 60 mins*	**Walk 9 miles (14.4km)** *about 126–135 mins + 15 mins stretch and strengthen*	**18 miles (28.8km)**
Day 81	**Day 82**	**Day 83**	**Day 84**	**Total**
Core stability training *for 60 mins*	**Walk 3 miles (4.8km)** *about 39–42 mins + 15 mins stretch and strengthen*	**Rest** *15 mins stretch and strengthen*	**Walk 10 miles (16km)** *about 140–150 mins + 15 mins stretch and strengthen*	**23 miles (36.8km)**

Key

- Walk days
- Other activity days
- Rest days

Exercise pages
- Warming up and cooling down, see Warm-up and cooldown plan p72 • Stretch and strengthen, see Stretching and strengthening plan p73 • Exercise-ball training, see pp56–59, p131, p139

ADVANCED: STAGE 1

This program is for walkers who wish to increase the intensity and distance of their walking. There are three stages to the program: the first builds stamina, the second focuses on speed, and the third works on stamina and speed together to help you achieve a high level of ability. Your aim at the end of the program is to walk 11–12 minutes per 1 mile (1.6km).

Before you start this program, you must be able to walk 1 mile (1.6km) in 15 minutes at a constant pace, and walk comfortably for 10 miles (16km) at a reasonable pace. You can return to any part of this program at any time and repeat weeks until you are ready to move on to the next stage.

Week 1–4

In these weeks, you are building stamina and strength with daily stretching, core stability exercises, and long-distance walking. Warm up and cool down for each walk. Stretching and strengthening is important because it helps you to walk at speed. To make the sequence fit the time specified, hold stretches for longer and include more repetitions on other exercises. Interval training is a good way to add variety to your walks. It does work the body quite hard, so have a rest day or an easy walk afterward. To add variety to your walks, you have the option of hill walking from week 3 onward. This means walking a route that takes you up and down hills.

	SUNDAY	MONDAY	TUESDAY
WEEK 1	**Day 1** **Walk 4 x 15-min miles** (6.4 x 10-min km) *about 60 mins*	**Day 2** **Core stability training** *for 60 mins*	**Day 3** **Walk 5 x15-min miles** (8 x 10-min km) *about 75 mins* *+ 15 mins stretch and strengthen*
WEEK 2	**Day 8** **Rest** *30 mins stretch and strengthen*	**Day 9** **Walk 6 x 15-min miles** (9.6 x 8–9-min km) *about 90 mins*	**Day 10** **Any other activity** *for 60 mins*
WEEK 3	**Day 15** **Rest** *30 mins stretch and strengthen*	**Day 16** **Walk 5 x 14–15-min miles** (8 x 10–11-min km) *about 70 mins* *+ 15 mins stretch and strengthen*	**Day 17** **Hill walking 7 x 15-min miles** (11.2 x 10-min km) *about 105 mins*
WEEK 4	**Day 22** **Walk 12 x 15-min miles** (19.2 x 10-min km) *about 180 mins* *+ 20 mins stretch and strengthen*	**Day 23** **Any other activity** *for 30 mins*	**Day 24** **Walk 5 x 15-min miles** (8 x 10-min km) *about 75 mins*

Other pages to help you
- Any other activity, see pp134-137 • Interval training, see pp110–111 • Hill walking, see pp112–113 • Staying injury-free, see pp126–131 • Foods for fitness, see pp90–91

This program sets you both a distance to walk and an ideal speed in which to complete it. If you walk to the speed suggested for each mile (or kilometer), you will progress quickly. However, always match the intensity of your walk to what you feel you can manage on a given day. A training walk can be exchanged for working with weights for 30 minutes or a walk on a treadmill if you wish, but not more than once a week. Adapt the program to suit your ability by using a heart-rate monitor to ensure you work at your peak. Add interest to your walks by using interval training combined with a heart-rate monitor. If time is short, concentrate on short distances and vary your speeds, or do interval training.

Key
- Walk days
- Other activity days
- Rest days

WEDNESDAY	THURSDAY	FRIDAY	SATURDAY	
Day 4 **Rest** *30 mins stretch and strengthen*	**Day 5** **Walk 6 x 15-min miles** **(9.6 x 10-min km)** *about 90 mins*	**Day 6** **Any other activity** *for 30 mins minimum*	**Day 7** **Walk 10 x 15-min miles** **(16 x 10-min km)** *about 150 mins*	**Total** **25 miles** **(40km)**
Day 11 **Walk 7 x 15-min miles** **(11.2 x 8–9-min km)** *about 105 mins*	**Day 12** **Interval training 4 miles** **(6.4km)** *about 56 mins*	**Day 13** **Walk 5 x 15-min miles** **(8 x 10-min km)** *about 75 mins + 15 mins stretch and strengthen*	**Day 14** **Walk 12 x 15-min miles** **(19.2 x 10-min km)** *about 180 mins*	**Total** **34 miles** **(54.4km)**
Day 18 **Any other activity** *for 60 mins*	**Day 19** **Walk 7 x 14–15-min miles** **(11.2 x 9–10-min km)** *about 98–105 mins + 15 mins stretch and strengthen*	**Day 20** **Walk 5 x 13–14-min miles** **(8 x 8–9-min km)** *about 65–70 mins + 20 mins stretch and strengthen*	**Day 21** **Swiss-ball training** *for 30 mins*	**Total** **24 miles** **(38.4km)**
Day 25 **Walk 7 x 13–14-min miles** **(11.2 x 8–9-min km)** *about 91–98 mins*	**Day 26** **Hill walking 6 miles** **(9.6km)** *about 90 mins*	**Day 27** **Walk 7 x 15-min miles** **(11.2 x 10-min km)** *about 105 mins + 20 mins stretch and strengthen*	**Day 28** **Swiss-ball training** *for 30 mins*	**Total** **37 miles** **(59.2km)**

Exercise pages
- Warming up and cooling down, see Warm-up and cooldown plan p72 • Core stability training, see pp54-59 • Stretch and strengthen, see Stretching and strengthening plan, see p73 • Swiss-ball training, see pp56-59, p131, p139

ADVANCED: STAGE 2

Weeks 5–8

The focus for the next 4 weeks is to work on shorter distances but increase the speed. It is advisable to keep to roads and pavements for this part of the plan.

The combination of walking, interval training, and core stability workouts provides no better way to increase overall body strength. By this part of the plan, you will already have a good base to work from.

Kettlebell training is an ideal discipline to include. It is based around four simple moves that are put together in endless combinations. Initially, it is advisable to join a class in order to receive instruction on handling a kettlebell and the correct technique. After that, you can easily do your sessions at home.

		SUNDAY	MONDAY	TUESDAY
WEEK 5		Day 29 **Walk 3 x 13–14-min miles** (4.8 x 10-min km) *about 42 mins*	Day 30 **Interval training 4 x 11–13-min miles** (6.4 x 7–8-min km) *about 44–52 mins*	Day 31 **Walk 2 x 15-min miles** (3.2 x 10-min km) *about 30 mins*
WEEK 6		Day 36 **Walk 3 x 13–14-min miles** (4.8 x 9–10-min km) *about 39–42 mins*	Day 37 **Interval training 4 x 11–13-min miles** (6.4 x 7–8-min km) *about 44–52 mins*	Day 38 **Core stability training** *for 30 mins*
WEEK 7		Day 43 **Walk 4 x 15-min miles** (6.4 x 10-min km) *about 60 mins*	Day 44 **Walk 6 x 13–14-min miles** (9.6 x 8–9-min km) *about 78–84 mins*	Day 45 **Interval training 2 x 11–13-min miles** (3.2 x 7–8-min km) *about 22–26 mins*
WEEK 8		Day 50 **Walk 2 x 13–14-min miles** (3.2 x 8–9min km) *about 26–28 mins*	Day 51 **Walk 3 x 15-min miles** (4.8 x 10-min km) *about 45 mins*	Day 52 **Interval training 4 x 11–13-min miles** (6.4 x 7–8-min km) *about 44–52 mins*

Other pages to help you
• Any other activity, see pp134-137 • Interval training, see pp110–111 • Hill walking, see pp112-113 • Staying injury-free, see pp126–131 • Foods for fitness, see pp90–91

WEDNESDAY	THURSDAY	FRIDAY	SATURDAY	
Day 32	**Day 33**	**Day 34**	**Day 35**	**Total**
Walk 2 x 3–14-min miles (3.2 x 9–10-min km) *about 26–28 mins*	**Core stability training** *for 30 mins*	**Interval training 4 x 11–13-min miles** (6.4 x 7–8-min km) *about 44–52 mins*	**Walk 5 x 15-min miles** (8 x 10-min km) *about 75 mins*	**20 miles** (32km)
Day 39	**Day 40**	**Day 41**	**Day 42**	**Total**
Walk 6 x 15-min miles (9.6 x 10-min km) *about 90 mins*	**Interval training 4 x 11–13-min miles** (6.4 x 7–8-min km) *about 44–52 mins*	**Walk 5 x 15-min miles** (8 x 10-min km) *about 75 mins*	**Walk 3 x 13–14-min miles** (4.8 x 9–10-min km) *about 39–42 mins*	**25 miles** (40km)
Day 46	**Day 47**	**Day 48**	**Day 49**	**Total**
Walk 5 x 15-min miles (8 x 10-min km) *about 75 mins*	**Core stability training** *for 30 mins*	**Walk 3 x 11–13-min miles** (6.4 x 8–9 min km) *about 33–39 mins*	**Walk 3 x 11–13-min miles** (4.8 x 7–8-min km) *about 33–39 mins*	**23 miles** (38.4km)
Day 53	**Day 54**	**Day 55**	**Day 56**	**Total**
Core stability training *for 30 mins*	**Interval training 2 x 13-min miles** (3.2 x 10-min km) *about 26 mins*	**Walk 3 x 15-min miles** (4.8 x 10-min km) *about 45 mins*	**Interval training 4 x 11–13-min miles** (6.4 x 7–8-min km) *about 44–52 mins*	**18 miles** (28.8km)

Key

- Walk days
- Other activity days
- Rest days

Exercise pages
- Warming up and cooling down, see Warm-up and cooldown plan p72   • Core stability training, see pp54-59   • Stretch and strengthen, see Stretching and strengthening plan p73
- Swiss-ball training, see pp56-59, p131, p139

ADVANCED: STAGE 3

Weeks 9–12

The final 4 weeks of the plan is a process of bringing together all the techniques and skills that you have worked on, to be able to power walk with speed and stamina.

When you have completed the plan you can use the program as a guide to continue increasing distance and speed as required. Make sure that you have a good variety of routes to keep you motivated.

If you feel you would like put your newfound fitness to the test, try orienteering. It's an adventure and endurance sport that brings together the balance between mental and physical exertion.

It promises great fun while giving you the opportunity to explore parts of the countryside that you would never normally see.

	SUNDAY	MONDAY	TUESDAY
WEEK 9	**Day 57** **Any other activity** *for 30 mins*	**Day 58** **Interval training 4 miles** (6.4km) *about 48–54 mins*	**Day 59** **Walk 6 x 11–13-min miles** (9.6 x 7–8-min km) *about 66–78 mins*
WEEK 10	**Day 64** **Walk 5 x 14-min miles** (8 x 9-min km) *about 70 mins* *+ 20 mins stretch and strengthen*	**Day 65** **Walk 7 x 12–14-min miles** (11.2 x 8–9-min km) *about 84–98 mins*	**Day 66** **Core stability training** *for 30 mins*
WEEK 11	**Day 71** **Walk 12 x 13–14-min miles** (19.2 x 8–10-min km) *about 156–168 mins* *+ 20 mins stretch and strengthen*	**Day 72** **Core stability training** *for 30 mins*	**Day 73** **Walk 3 x 11-min miles** (4.8 x 7-min km) *about 33 mins* *+ 20 mins stretch and strengthen*
WEEK 12	**Day 78** **Walk 4 x 15-min miles** (6.4 x 10-min km) *about 60 mins*	**Day 79** **Walk 5 x 11–13-min miles** (8 x 7–8-min km) *about 55–56 mins* *+ 15 mins stretch and strengthen*	**Day 80** **Any other activity** *for 60 mins*

Other pages to help you
- Any other activity, see pp134-137 • Interval training, see pp110–111 • Hill walking, see pp112-113 • Staying injury-free, see pp126-131 • Foods for fitness, see pp90–91

WEDNESDAY	THURSDAY	FRIDAY	SATURDAY	
Day 60	**Day 61**	**Day 62**	**Day 63**	**Total**
Core stability training *for 30 mins*	**Walk 3 x 13-min miles** (4.8 x 8-min km) *about 36 mins*	**Hill walking 4 miles** (6.4km) *about 52–60 mins*	**Walk 10 x 13–15-min miles** (16 x 9–10-min km) *about 130–150 mins*	**27 miles** (43.2km)
Day 67	**Day 68**	**Day 69**	**Day 70**	**Total**
Any other activity *for 60 mins*	**Hill walking 4 miles** (6.4km) *about 48–52 mins + 15 mins stretch and strengthen*	**Interval training 6 miles** (9.6km) *about 78–84 mins + 20 mins stretch and strengthen*	**Walk 7 x 12–14-min miles** (11.2 x 7–8-min km) *about 84–98 mins + 15 mins stretch and strengthen*	**29 miles** (46.4km)
Day 74	**Day 75**	**Day 76**	**Day 77**	**Total**
Walk 5 x 14-min miles (8 x 9-min km) *about 70 mins + 15 mins stretch and strengthen*	**Any other activity** *for 30 mins*	**Walk 6 x 11–13-min miles** (9.6 x 8-min km) *about 66–78 mins + 20 mins stretch and strengthen*	**Hill walking 10 x 13–14-min miles** (16 x 8–9-min km) *about 130–140 mins*	**36 miles** (57.6km)
Day 81	**Day 82**	**Day 83**	**Day 84**	**Total**
Interval training 3 miles (4.8 km) *about 33–39 mins*	**Core stability training** *for 30 mins*	**Walk 5 x 15-min miles** (8 x 10-min km) *about 75 mins + 15 mins stretch and strengthen*	**Walk 12 x 11–13-min miles** (19.2 x 7–8-min km) *about 132–143 mins*	**29 miles** (46.4km)

Key

■ Walk days

□ Other activity days

□ Rest days

Exercise pages
• Warming up and cooling down, see Warm-up and cooldown plan p72 • Core stability training, see pp54-59 • Stretch and strengthen, see Stretching and strengthening plan p73
• Swiss-ball training, see pp56-59, p131, p139

SHORT DISTANCE: STAGE 1

The aim of this program is to help you reach a level of fitness that allows you to power walk for 1 hour a day. Before you begin, you must be able to walk for 15 minutes at any speed. If this is uncomfortable for you, try the beginner program (pp140–145) until you reach this level of ability.

Week 1

Start with a steady pace; speed is not important. Allow your body to adapt to the idea of walking every day and notice how your body feels. Warm up before each walk by stretching 5 minutes into the beginning of your walk, and cool down by slowing for the last 10 minutes of your walk and stretching immediately after. Reduce the amount of time on warm-up and cooldown stretches on shorter walks of 30 minutes or less.

Week 2

If you are ready, use more exertion. You should feel that your body is working harder (a heart-rate monitor will give you a more accurate measurement of how hard), but you should be able to talk as you walk.

Weeks 3–4

By now, you should feel you have more energy. If you are comfortable with the length of time you are walking, start to increase your speed further.

	SUNDAY	MONDAY	TUESDAY
WEEK 1	Day 1 15 minutes	Day 2 15 minutes	Day 3 15 minutes
WEEK 2	Day 8 20 minutes	Day 9 15 minutes	Day 10 20 minutes
WEEK 3	Day 15 20 minutes	Day 16 15 minutes	Day 17 20 minutes
WEEK 4	Day 22 20 minutes	Day 23 25 minutes	Day 24 20 minutes

Other pages to help you
• Using a pedometer, see pp36–37 • Using a heart-rate monitor, see pp32–35 • Interval training, see pp110–111 • Posture and breathing, see pp40–41 • Fit walking into your day, see pp94–95

As a guide, 1 mile (1.6km) in 15 minutes is a good pace for you to aim at. The average person walks 2½–3 miles (2.4–4.8km) per hour, and your aim by the end of this 12-week program is to walk at about 4 miles (6.4km) per hour. This table is based on minutes walked, not distance. By completing short distances regularly, your stamina and speed will increase simultaneously. Success is guaranteed if you power walk at least four times a week and exert yourself for the specified period of time. Daily walks of a minimum of 30 minutes could be split into two 15-minute walks so that the program can fit your life more easily.

Key
- Walk days
- Other activity days
- Rest days

WEDNESDAY	THURSDAY	FRIDAY	SATURDAY	
Day 4	Day 5	Day 6	Day 7	Total
20 minutes	15 minutes	15 minutes	15 minutes	110 minutes
Day 11	Day 12	Day 13	Day 14	Total
15 minutes	15 minutes	15 minutes	15 minutes	115 minutes
Day 18	Day 19	Day 20	Day 21	Total
20 minutes	15 minutes	25 minutes	20 minutes	135 minutes
Day 25	Day 26	Day 27	Day 28	Total
20 minutes	25 minutes	25 minutes	30 minutes	165 minutes

Exercise pages
- Warming up and cooling down, see Warm-up and cooldown plan p72 • Stretch and strengthen, see Stretching and strengthening plan p73

SHORT DISTANCE: STAGE 2

Weeks 5–8

From week 5, the walking time is beginning to increase, as well as your speed. Apart from having favorite walks, make sure that you continually plot new ones to keep you motivated, taking into account that you will continue to walk farther within the same time period.

This is also a good time to try out interval training. Try walking as fast as you can for 30 seconds to 1 minute, and then relax the speed and walk more slowly to recover for double the amount of time (so 1–2 minutes). You can repeat this again four or five times, or as often as you feel able within a session. Be aware it is very intense, and should not be repeated on two training days in a row.

Working on your technique is another way to increase speed. Make sure you have good posture with your shoulders down and back, and your pelvis just slightly tipped forward, even if you have not yet reached a speed where you are using your arms to propel you forward. It is useful to hold them in the right position, at right angles at your sides, for when you do use them.

	SUNDAY	MONDAY	TUESDAY
WEEK 5	Day 29 **20 minutes**	Day 30 **20 minutes**	Day 31 **25 minutes**
WEEK 6	Day 36 **25 minutes**	Day 37 **30 minutes**	Day 38 **30 minutes**
WEEK 7	Day 43 **25 minutes**	Day 44 **30 minutes**	Day 45 **40 minutes**
WEEK 8	Day 50 **30 minutes**	Day 51 **35 minutes**	Day 52 **40 minutes**

Other pages to help you
• Using a pedometer, see pp36–37 • Using a heart-rate monitor, see pp32–35 • Interval training, see pp110–111 • Posture and breathing, see pp40–41 • Fit walking into your day, see pp94–95

WEDNESDAY	THURSDAY	FRIDAY	SATURDAY	
Day 32	**Day 33**	**Day 34**	**Day 35**	**Total**
30 minutes	**20 minutes**	**25 minutes**	**30 minutes**	**170 minutes**
Day 39	**Day 40**	**Day 41**	**Day 42**	**Total**
25 minutes	**30 minutes**	**30 minutes**	**35 minutes**	**205 minutes**
Day 46	**Day 47**	**Day 48**	**Day 49**	**Total**
25 minutes	**30 minutes**	**40 minutes**	**40 minutes**	**230 minutes**
Day 53	**Day 54**	**Day 55**	**Day 56**	**Total**
30 minutes	**35 minutes**	**40 minutes**	**40 minutes**	**250 minutes**

Key

- Walk days
- Other activity days
- Rest days

Exercise pages
- Warming up and cooling down, see Warm-up and cooldown plan p72 • Stretch and strengthen, see Stretching and strengthening plan p73

SHORT DISTANCE: STAGE 3

Weeks 9–12

It is a great feeling to experience yourself getting fitter and stronger. With the right technique, walking can achieve a total-body workout like nothing else. In these last weeks of the training plan, you should be feeling much more confident in your walking as you reach your goal of walking an hour daily.

There is no reason that you should stop when you reach week 12; however, you may want to set yourself a new goal or challenge. Or you can continue with your daily hour and look for creative ways to keep your challenge fresh. Find new routes and terrains, speed challenges, and walking meditations, or even form a group to walk with friends. Nordic walking is also a fun workout for short-distance walkers. It can present a different experience to power walking, particularly if you go off-road. Join a class, and not only will you have walking companions, but you will also probably find the instructor will provide the poles.

You may also enjoy the challenge of 10,000 steps a day. By using a fitness tracker or device, you can include a possible 10,000 steps a day into your daily hour of walking.

	SUNDAY	**MONDAY**	**TUESDAY**
WEEK 9	Day 57 30 minutes	Day 58 40 minutes	Day 59 40 minutes
WEEK 10	Day 64 30 minutes	Day 65 40 minutes	Day 66 50 minutes
WEEK 11	Day 71 30 minutes	Day 72 40 minutes	Day 73 50 minutes
WEEK 12	Day 78 40 minutes	Day 79 50 minutes	Day 80 60 minutes

Other pages to help you
• Using a pedometer, see pp36–37 • Using a heart-rate monitor, see pp32–35 • Interval training, see pp110–111 • Posture and breathing, see pp40–41 • Fit walking into your day, see pp94–95

WEDNESDAY	THURSDAY	FRIDAY	SATURDAY	
Day 60	**Day 61**	**Day 62**	**Day 63**	**Total**
30 minutes	**30 minutes**	**30 minutes**	**50 minutes**	**250 minutes**
Day 67	**Day 68**	**Day 69**	**Day 70**	**Total**
30 minutes	**40 minutes**	**40 minutes**	**50 minutes**	**280 minutes**
Day 74	**Day 75**	**Day 76**	**Day 77**	**Total**
30 minutes	**30 minutes**	**50 minutes**	**60 minutes**	**290 minutes**
Day 81	**Day 82**	**Day 83**	**Day 84**	**Total**
30 minutes	**40 minutes**	**50 minutes**	**60 minutes**	**330 minutes**

Key

Walk days

Other activity days

Rest days

Exercise pages
- Warming up and cooling down, see Warm-up and cooldown plan p72 • Stretch and strengthen, see Stretching and strengthening plan p73

HALF-MARATHON: STAGE 1

To begin this program, you must be able to walk 2 miles (3.2km) at a constant speed of approximately 18–20 minutes per 1 mile (1.6km). If you are unable to do this, try the beginner program (pp140–145) until you are able to achieve this pace. By the end of the half-marathon program, your aim is to be walking at a speed of 14–15 minutes per 1 mile (1.6km).

A good finishing time for a half-marathon is 2¾–3 hours.

Weeks 1–2

Start with a steady pace and pay particular attention to your posture and technique. A steady pace means you do not need to push yourself hard. Warm up before each walk by stretching 5 minutes into the beginning of your walk, and cool down by slowing for the last 10 minutes of your walk and stretching immediately after. On your rest days, stretch and strengthen for at least 10 minutes, or longer if you would prefer, using the daily stretching and strengthening plan.

Weeks 3–4

Any other activity can be anything you choose for a minimum of 15 minutes that increases your heart rate, such as swimming, dancing, or rollerblading. You are now walking at a faster pace, which means you are walking with purpose and that you are exerting yourself, but you should still able to talk as you walk.

	SUNDAY	MONDAY	TUESDAY
WEEK 1	Day 1 **Walk 2 miles (3.2km) at a steady pace** *about 40 mins*	Day 2 **Rest** *10–15 mins stretch and strengthen*	Day 3 **Walk 2 miles (3.2km) at a steady pace** *about 40 mins*
WEEK 2	Day 8 **Rest** *10–15 mins stretch and strengthen*	Day 9 **Walk 2 miles (3.2km) at a steady pace** *about 36 mins*	Day 10 **Rest** *10–15 mins stretch and strengthen*
WEEK 3	Day 15 **Rest** *10–15 mins stretch and strengthen*	Day 16 **Walk 3 miles (4.8km) at a faster pace** *about 54 mins*	Day 17 **Any other activity** *for a minimum of 30 mins*
WEEK 4	Day 22 **Rest** *10–15 mins stretch and strengthen*	Day 23 **Walk 3 miles (4.8km) at a faster pace** *about 54 mins*	Day 24 **Any other activity** *for a minimum of 30 mins*

Other pages to help you
- Foods for fitness, see pp90–91 • Preparing for a marathon, see pp106–107 • Using a heart-rate monitor, see pp32–35 • Any other activity, see pp134–137

Use this program as a guide only and adapt it to suit your level of fitness and your life. The goal is to achieve a good, constantly maintained speed over 13.2 miles (21.1km), the distance of a half-marathon. The program starts with walks at a steady pace over longer distances to build stamina and strength. When you feel ready, pick up the pace to work on your speed. Use the times given here as approximate goals for which you should aim. It takes 4–6 weeks for your body to fully adapt to any cardiovascular change—too fast, too soon can cause injuries. Eventually, you will find that speed and stamina will come together.

Key

Walk days

Other activity days

Rest days

WEDNESDAY	**THURSDAY**	**FRIDAY**	**SATURDAY**	
Day 4	Day 5	Day 6	Day 7	Total
Rest *10–15 mins stretch and strengthen*	**Walk 2 miles (3.2km) at a steady pace** *about 40 mins*	**Rest** *10–15 mins stretch and strengthen*	**Walk 3 miles (4.8km) at a steady pace** *about 60 mins*	**9 miles (14.4km)**
Day 11	Day 12	Day 13	Day 14	Total
Walk 3 miles (4.8km) at a steady pace *about 54 mins*	**Rest** *10–15 mins stretch and strengthen*	**Rest** *10–15 mins stretch and strengthen*	**Walk 3 miles (4.8km) at a steady pace** *about 54 mins*	**8 miles (12.8km)**
Day 18	Day 19	Day 20	Day 21	Total
Walk 4 miles (6.4km) at a steady pace *about 80 mins*	**Rest** *10–15 mins stretch and strengthen*	**Any other activity** *for a minimum of 30 mins*	**Walk 5 miles (8km) at a steady pace** *about 100 mins*	**12 miles (19.2km)**
Day 25	Day 26	Day 27	Day 28	Total
Walk 3 miles (4.8km) at a faster pace *about 50 mins*	**Rest** *10–15 mins stretch and strengthen*	**Walk 3 miles (4.8km) at a faster pace** *about 50 mins*	**Rest** *10–15 mins stretch and strengthen*	**9 miles (14.4km)**

Exercise pages
• Warming up and cooling down, see Warm-up and cooldown plan p72 • Stretch and strengthen, see Stretching and strengthening plan p73

HALF-MARATHON: STAGE 2

Weeks 5–8

By week 5, you will be ready to begin exerting yourself more on the short walks. Try increasing your pace, but at the same time keeping it constant. Make sure that even though you are increasing your heart rate, you can still hold a conversation. This all takes practice, but keep going; you have come a long way.

Meanwhile, it is better to walk at a slightly slower pace on your longer walks, but again work at keeping it constant. This will develop your endurance and eventually the speed of your shorter walks will link up with the stamina and endurance that you have developed on the long walks.

By now you should also be enjoying your other activities. You do not necessarily need to stick to the same ones throughout your training; however, continuity does help when it comes to sticking to a schedule or planning your week.

Don't forget that rest and stretch days are just as important as walking days. Stretching regularly will help you to reach the finish line comfortably, having enjoyed the whole experience.

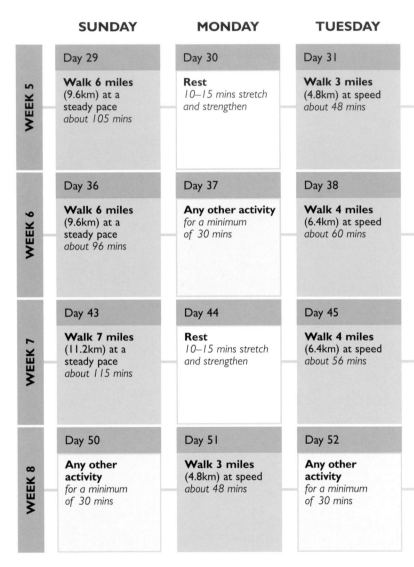

	SUNDAY	MONDAY	TUESDAY
WEEK 5	Day 29 **Walk 6 miles** (9.6km) at a steady pace *about 105 mins*	Day 30 **Rest** *10–15 mins stretch and strengthen*	Day 31 **Walk 3 miles** (4.8km) at speed *about 48 mins*
WEEK 6	Day 36 **Walk 6 miles** (9.6km) at a steady pace *about 96 mins*	Day 37 **Any other activity** *for a minimum of 30 mins*	Day 38 **Walk 4 miles** (6.4km) at speed *about 60 mins*
WEEK 7	Day 43 **Walk 7 miles** (11.2km) at a steady pace *about 115 mins*	Day 44 **Rest** *10–15 mins stretch and strengthen*	Day 45 **Walk 4 miles** (6.4km) at speed *about 56 mins*
WEEK 8	Day 50 **Any other activity** *for a minimum of 30 mins*	Day 51 **Walk 3 miles** (4.8km) at speed *about 48 mins*	Day 52 **Any other activity** *for a minimum of 30 mins*

Other pages to help you

• Foods for fitness, see pp90–91 • Preparing for a marathon, see pp106–107 • Using a heart-rate monitor, see pp32–35 • Any other activity, see pp134–137

WEDNESDAY	THURSDAY	FRIDAY	SATURDAY	
Day 32 **Any other activity** *for a minimum of 30 mins*	**Day 33** **Walk 4 miles (6.4km) at a steady pace** *about 60–64 mins*	**Day 34** **Rest** *10–15 mins stretch and strengthen*	**Day 35** **Any other activity** *for a minimum of 30 mins*	**Total** **13 miles (20.8km)**
Day 39 **Rest** *10–15 mins stretch and strengthen*	**Day 40** **Walk 4 miles (6.4km) at speed** *about 60 mins*	**Day 41** **Any other activity** *for a minimum of 30 mins*	**Day 42** **Rest** *10–15 mins stretch and strengthen*	**Total** **14 miles (22.4km)**
Day 46 **Rest** *10–15 mins stretch and strengthen*	**Day 47** **Walk 4 miles (6.4km) at speed** *about 56 mins*	**Day 48** **Rest** *10–15 mins stretch and strengthen*	**Day 49** **Walk 5 miles (8km) at a steady pace** *about 80 mins*	**Total** **20 miles (32km)**
Day 53 **Walk 3 miles (4.8km) at speed** *about 42 mins*	**Day 54** **Any other activity** *for a minimum of 30 mins*	**Day 55** **Walk 3 miles (4.8km) at speed** *about 42 mins*	**Day 56** **Rest** *10–15 mins stretch and strengthen*	**Total** **9 miles (14.4km)**

Key

- Walk days
- Other activity days
- Rest days

Exercise pages
- Warming up and cooling down, see Warm-up and cooldown plan p72 • Stretch and strengthen, see Stretching and strengthening plan p73

HALF-MARATHON: STAGE 3

Weeks 9–12
By the last 4 weeks of your training, you may have surprised yourself at how far you have come and how different you feel as a result of regular walking.

These last few weeks are split between reaching the climax of your training and then resting in preparation of the challenge. In week 11, you will complete a 10-mile (16km) training walk. Completing this distance really is a landmark moment in your training. It will probably be the farthest you have walked, but will ensure that if you can walk 10 miles (16km), you can most certainly reach the finish line. This is a very special moment for anyone, but particularly if you have never attempted a challenge like this before.

Don't forget that once you complete your distance, your body will have been put under a certain amount of stress and will require a little loving care. Make sure that you have some warm clothes to put on, and that you have access to hot food, like porridge or soup, or that you take food with you. A snack of carbs or protein will help to replenish your blood sugar levels and go toward repairing muscle tissue.

Keep walking slowly, whether it be to a bus, train, or car, as this will help to release the lactic acid. It is, of course, also helpful to do some stretches!

	SUNDAY	MONDAY	TUESDAY
WEEK 9	Day 57 **Walk 8 miles** (12.9km) at speed *about 120 mins*	Day 58 **Rest** *10–15 mins stretch and strengthen*	Day 59 **Walk 4 miles** (6.4km) at speed *about 56–60 mins*
WEEK 10	Day 64 **Rest** *10–15 mins stretch and strengthen*	Day 65 **Any other activity** *for a minimum of 30 mins*	Day 66 **Walk 4 miles** (6.4km) at speed *about 55–60 mins*
WEEK 11	Day 71 **Walk 10 miles** (16km) at speed *about 140 mins*	Day 72 **Rest** *10–15 mins stretch and strengthen*	Day 73 **Rest** *10–15 mins stretch and strengthen*
WEEK 12	Day 78 **Rest** *10–15 mins stretch and strengthen*	Day 79 **Any other activity** *for a minimum of 30 mins*	Day 80 **Rest** *10–15 mins stretch and strengthen*

Other pages to help you
• Foods for fitness, see pp90–91 • Preparing for a marathon, see pp106–107 • Using a heart-rate monitor, see pp32–35 • Any other activity, see pp134–137

WEDNESDAY	THURSDAY	FRIDAY	SATURDAY	
Day 60	**Day 61**	**Day 62**	**Day 63**	**Total**
Rest *10–15 mins stretch and strengthen*	**Walk 4 miles (6.4km) at speed** *about 55–60 mins*	**Any other activity** *for a minimum of 30 mins*	**Walk 8 miles (12.9km) at speed** *about 112 mins*	**24 miles (38.6km)**
Day 67	**Day 68**	**Day 69**	**Day 70**	**Total**
Rest *10–15 mins stretch and strengthen*	**Walk 4 miles (6.4km) at speed** *about 55–60 mins*	**Any other activity** *for a minimum of 30 mins*	**Rest** *10–15 mins stretch and strengthen*	**8 miles (12.8km)**
Day 74	**Day 75**	**Day 76**	**Day 77**	**Total**
Walk 3 miles (4.8km) at speed *about 40–43 mins*	**Any other activity** *for a minimum of 30 mins*	**Rest** *10–15 mins stretch and strengthen*	**Walk 3 miles (4.8km) at speed** *about 40–43 mins*	**16 miles (25.6km)**
Day 81	**Day 82**	**Day 83**	**Day 84**	**Total**
Walk 3 miles (4.8km) at speed *about 40 mins*	**Rest** *10–15 mins stretch and strengthen*	**Walk 3 miles (4.8km) at speed** *about 40 mins*	**Rest** *10–15 mins stretch and strengthen*	**6 miles (9.6km)**

Key

Walk days

Other activity days

Rest days

Exercise pages
- Warming up and cooling down, see Warm-up and cooldown plan p72 • Stretch and strengthen, see Stretching and strengthening plan p73

MARATHON: STAGE 1

Marathoners take on the challenge for many reasons, from wanting to conquer a personal goal to raising money for charity. Whatever the aim, everybody wants that magical moment of crossing the finish line. Preparation is the key to success, and by following this 12-week program, there is no reason the magic cannot be yours.

A good finishing time for a marathon (26¼ miles/42.2km) is 6 hours. The aim is to walk at a constant speed of 12–14 minutes per 1 mile (1.6km).

Weeks 1–2

Work on your technique and posture in these first weeks and walk at a comfortable and constant pace, but make sure that you can feel an increase in your heart rate and that you are exerting yourself beyond your normal pace. However, going too fast too soon can cause injuries, so focus on a constant pace over speed. Warm up and cool down for each walk. On the days when you are not walking, set aside time for stretching and strengthening. Start with a session of around 10 minutes and extend this as time goes on.

Week 3

You need to be walking at a faster pace now, which means exerting yourself, but ensure you are still able to talk as you walk. The other activity can be anything you enjoy, such as swimming, dancing, or orienteering.

Week 4

Start increasing your pace, and introduce interval training into your mid-week sessions. Interval training works the body quite hard, so have a rest day or an easy walk afterward.

	SUNDAY	MONDAY	TUESDAY
WEEK 1	**Day 1** **Walk 3 miles** (4.8km) at a comfortable pace *about 55–60 mins*	**Day 2** **Rest** *10–15 mins stretch and strengthen*	**Day 3** **Walk 3 miles** (4.8km) at a comfortable pace *about 55–60 mins*
WEEK 2	**Day 8** **Walk 4 miles** (6.4km) at a comfortable pace *about 72–80 mins*	**Day 9** **Rest** *10–15 mins stretch and strengthen*	**Day 10** **Walk 4 miles** (6.4km) at a comfortable pace *about 72–80 mins*
WEEK 3	**Day 15** **Walk 5 miles** (8km) at a comfortable pace *about 85–90 mins*	**Day 16** **Rest** *10–15 mins stretch and strengthen*	**Day 17** **Walk 4 miles** (6.4km) at a comfortable pace *about 68 mins*
WEEK 4	**Day 22** **Rest** *10–15 mins stretch and strengthen*	**Day 23** **Walk 5 miles** (8km) at a comfortable pace *about 85 mins*	**Day 24** **Any other activity** *for a minimum of 30 mins*

Other pages to help you
- Foods for fitness, see pp90–91 • Preparing for a marathon, see pp106–107 • Any other activity, see pp134–137 • Interval training, see pp110–111 • Using a pedometer, see pp36–37 • Using a heart-rate monitor, see pp32–35 • Meeting the challenge, see pp80–81

For this program, you must be able to walk 3 miles (4.8km) at a steady speed of approximately 18–20 minutes per 1 mile (1.6 km). If you are unable to do this, follow the beginner program until you can achieve this pace, then return to this program. If you need to train on a treadmill because of time restraints or lack of daylight hours, ensure that at least 50 percent of your training is on roads. Use the times given here as approximate goals for which you should aim.

Key

Walk days

Other activity days

Rest days

WEDNESDAY	THURSDAY	FRIDAY	SATURDAY	
Day 4	**Day 5**	**Day 6**	**Day 7**	**Total**
Rest *10–15 mins stretch and strengthen*	**Walk 3 miles (4.8km) at a comfortable pace** *about 55–60 mins*	**Rest** *10–15 mins stretch and strengthen*	**Rest** *10–15 mins stretch and strengthen*	**9 miles (14.4km)**
Day 11	**Day 12**	**Day 13**	**Day 14**	**Total**
Rest *10–15 mins stretch and strengthen*	**Walk 4 miles (6.4km) at a comfortable pace** *about 72–85 mins*	**Rest** *10–15 mins stretch and strengthen*	**Rest** *10–15 mins stretch and strengthen*	**12 miles (19.2km)**
Day 18	**Day 19**	**Day 20**	**Day 21**	**Total**
Any other activity *for a minimum of 30 mins*	**Walk 4 miles (6.4km) at a comfortable pace** *about 68 mins*	**Rest** *10–15 mins stretch and strengthen*	**Walk 6 miles (9.6km) at a comfortable pace** *about 102 mins*	**19 miles (30.4km)**
Day 25	**Day 26**	**Day 27**	**Day 28**	**Total**
Interval training 5 miles (8km) *about 85 mins*	**Any other activity** *for a minimum of 30 mins*	**Rest** *10–15 mins stretch and strengthen*	**Walk 8 miles (12.9km) at a comfortable pace** *about 136 mins*	**18 miles (28.9km)**

Exercise pages
• Stretching exercises, see pp60–67 • Warming up and cooling down, see Warm-up and cooldown plan p72 • Exercise-ball training, see pp56–59, p131, p139

MARATHON: STAGE 2

Weeks 5–8

By week 5, you should be feeling the rhythm of your walk, along with the benefits of regular exercise. Make sure that your device is tracking your progress, as each stepping stone of success empowers you to go forward.

Introduce some interval training as often as you wish. Alternate between walking as fast as you can for 1–2 minutes and then slowing down to recover for double the time of your fast walk (in other words, 2–4 minutes). This can be repeated as often as you wish within a session, although it can be intense, so begin with 20–30 minutes.

	SUNDAY	MONDAY	TUESDAY
WEEK 5	Day 29 **Any other activity** *for a minimum of 30 mins*	Day 30 **Interval training 5 miles** **(8km)** *about 80 mins*	Day 31 **Rest** *10–15 mins stretch and strengthen*
WEEK 6	Day 36 **Rest** *10–15 mins stretch and strengthen*	Day 37 **Any other activity** *for a minimum of 30 mins*	Day 38 **Walk 4 miles (6.4km) at a faster pace** *about 60–64 mins*
WEEK 7	Day 43 **Rest** *10–15 mins stretch and strengthen*	Day 44 **Walk 6 miles (9.6km) at a faster pace** *about 90 mins*	Day 45 **Any other activity** *for a minimum of 30 mins*
WEEK 8	Day 50 **Walk 14 miles (22.5km) at a faster pace** *about 120 mins*	Day 51 **Rest** *10–15 mins stretch and strengthen*	Day 52 **Interval training 6 miles (9.6km)** *about 90–95 mins*

Other pages to help you
• Foods for fitness, see pp90–91 • Preparing for a marathon, see pp106–107 • Any other activity, see pp134–137 • Interval training, see pp110–111 • Using a pedometer, see pp36–37 • Using a heart-rate monitor, see pp32–35 • Meeting the challenge, see pp80–81

WEDNESDAY	THURSDAY	FRIDAY	SATURDAY	
Day 32 **Walk 5 miles** (8km) at a faster pace *about 75–80 mins*	**Day 33** **Any other activity** *for a minimum* *of 30 mins*	**Day 34** **Rest** *10–15 mins stretch* *and strengthen*	**Day 35** **Walk 10 miles** (16km) at a faster pace *about 160 mins*	**Total** **20 miles** (32km)
Day 39 **Any other activity** *for a minimum* *of 30 mins*	**Day 40** **Interval training** **6 miles** (9.6km) *about 75–80 mins*	**Day 41** **Rest** *10–15 mins stretch* *and strengthen*	**Day 42** **Walk 12 miles** (19.2km) at a faster pace *about 180–192 mins*	**Total** **22 miles** (35.2km)
Day 46 **Rest** *10–15 mins stretch* *and strengthen*	**Day 47** **Interval training** **6 miles** (9.6km) *about 90 mins*	**Day 48** **Any other activity** *for a minimum* *of 30 mins*	**Day 49** **Rest** *10–15 mins stretch* *and strengthen*	**Total** **12 miles** (19.2km)
Day 53 **Rest** *10–15 mins stretch* *and strengthen*	**Day 54** **Walk 6 miles** (9.6km) at a faster pace *about 90 mins*	**Day 55** **Rest** *10–15 mins stretch* *and strengthen*	**Day 56** **Walk 16 miles** (25.7km) at a faster pace *about 240 mins*	**Total** **42 miles** (67.4km)

Key

■ Walk days
□ Other activity days
□ Rest days

Exercise pages
• Stretching exercises, see pp60–67 • Warming up and cooling down, see Warm-up and cooldown plan p72 • Exercise-ball training, see pp56–59, p131, p139

MARATHON: STAGE 3

Weeks 9–12

In the final four weeks of the plan, you will not only reach the climax of your training, but also go into the rest period following your 20-mile (32km) walk, allowing your body time to recover prior to the challenge.

Walking the 20-mile (32km) distance is an important part of the plan, both mentally and physically. If you can complete this distance, you will know you can reach the finish line.

If you have not done so already, take the opportunity in these last few weeks to eat well, stay well hydrated, and commit to spending time each day stretching. This level of preparation will contribute to how well supported your body feels on the day.

Don't forget that postevent care is also important. Your body will probably have been running on adrenaline for quite some time. As soon as you cross the finish line, eat carbohydrates and proteins to replenish your blood sugar levels and muscle glycogen, and to help repair muscle tissue. Soup is comforting if it is cold. Otherwise, porridge, a peanut butter sandwich, or yogurt with cereal are all good choices.

Make sure you have something warm to put on. Although you may not feel like it, slowly keep walking to release the lactic acid from your muscles. Of course, stretching on the day and subsequent days following the challenge is a must!

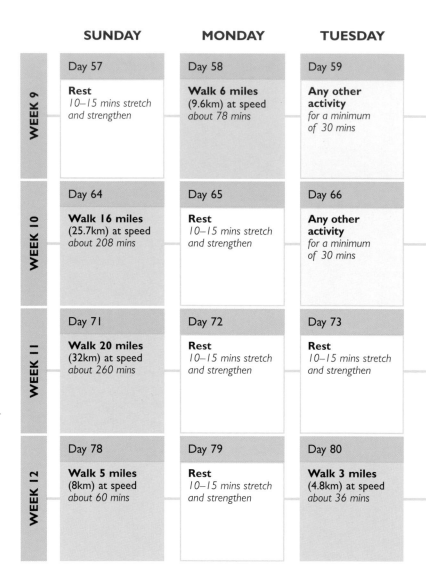

	SUNDAY	MONDAY	TUESDAY
WEEK 9	Day 57 **Rest** *10–15 mins stretch and strengthen*	Day 58 **Walk 6 miles** **(9.6km) at speed** *about 78 mins*	Day 59 **Any other activity** *for a minimum of 30 mins*
WEEK 10	Day 64 **Walk 16 miles** **(25.7km) at speed** *about 208 mins*	Day 65 **Rest** *10–15 mins stretch and strengthen*	Day 66 **Any other activity** *for a minimum of 30 mins*
WEEK 11	Day 71 **Walk 20 miles** **(32km) at speed** *about 260 mins*	Day 72 **Rest** *10–15 mins stretch and strengthen*	Day 73 **Rest** *10–15 mins stretch and strengthen*
WEEK 12	Day 78 **Walk 5 miles** **(8km) at speed** *about 60 mins*	Day 79 **Rest** *10–15 mins stretch and strengthen*	Day 80 **Walk 3 miles** **(4.8km) at speed** *about 36 mins*

Other pages to help you

• Foods for fitness, see pp90–91 • Preparing for a marathon, see pp106–107 • Any other activity, see pp134–137 • Interval training, see pp110–111 • Using a pedometer, see pp36–37 • Using a heart-rate monitor, see pp32–35 • Meeting the challenge, see pp80–81

WEDNESDAY	THURSDAY	FRIDAY	SATURDAY	
Day 60 **Interval training 7 miles** (11.2km) *about 90 mins*	Day 61 **Any other activity** *for a minimum of 30 mins*	Day 62 **Walk 6 miles** (9.6km) at speed *about 78–84 mins*	Day 63 **Rest** *10–15 mins stretch and strengthen*	Total **19 miles** (30.4km)
Day 67 **Interval training 7 miles** (11.2km) *about 90–100 mins*	Day 68 **Rest** *10–15 mins stretch and strengthen*	Day 69 **Walk 7 miles** (11.2km) at speed *about 90 mins*	Day 70 **Rest** *10–15 mins stretch and strengthen*	Total **30 miles** (48km)
Day 74 **Walk 5 miles** (8km) at speed *about 60 mins*	Day 75 **Rest** *10–15 mins stretch and strengthen*	Day 76 **Walk 5 miles** (8km) at speed *about 60 mins*	Day 77 **Any other activity** *for a minimum of 30 mins*	Total **30 miles** (48km)
Day 81 **Rest** *10–15 mins stretch and strengthen*	Day 82 **Walk 3 miles** (4.8km) at speed *about 36 mins*	Day 83 **Rest** *10–15 mins stretch and strengthen*	Day 84 **Rest** *10–15 mins stretch and strengthen*	Total **11 miles** (17.6km)

Key

- Walk days
- Other activity days
- Rest days

Exercise pages
- Stretching exercises, see pp60–67 • Warming up and cooling down, see Warm-up and cooldown plan p72 • Exercise-ball training, see pp56–59, p131, p139

WEIGHT LOSS: STAGE 1

To lose weight and burn calories, you must walk briskly for 45 minutes a minimum of four times a week. How many calories you will burn is dependent on several factors: your age, weight, level of fitness, and how fast and far you actually walk within the time. Your aim is to walk 1 mile (1.6km) in 15–17 minutes.

Walking will help you to lose weight, but you need to combine it with a healthy diet to ensure you achieve good and long-lasting results. If you are not used to any physical activity and unsure of your health and ability, please seek medical advice before starting this program. It is worth investing in a wearable device or fitness tracker that includes a calorie function. Depending on the technology and the model, you may also be able to measure and record weight, body fat percentage, and BMI. There are also apps and databases that hold the nutritional data and calorie content of foods.

Weeks 1–4

Beginning to walk at a steady pace means that you will probably be walking more energetically than usual. You should be aiming to walk for 20 minutes per 1 mile (1.6km). It's important to feel an increase in your heart rate, but you should still be able to talk while walking.

If you're finding the distance challenging, try walking with Nordic poles. The poles offer an element of support. Although you will probably move faster using the poles than not, the effort seems easier, and this may be just the motivation that works for you in the first few weeks.

Make time to regularly stretch, both before and after your walk, and on your rest days.

	SUNDAY	**MONDAY**	**TUESDAY**
WEEK 1	Day 1 **Walk** at a steady pace *for 10 mins*	Day 2 **Walk** at a steady pace *for 10 mins*	Day 3 **Walk** at a steady pace *for 10 mins*
WEEK 2	Day 8 **Walk** at a steady pace *for 15 mins*	Day 9 **Walk** at a steady pace *for 10 mins*	Day 10 **Walk** at a steady pace *for 15 mins* *+ any other activity* *for 30 mins*
WEEK 3	Day 15 **Walk** at a faster pace *for 20 mins*	Day 16 **Walk** at a faster pace *for 15 mins*	Day 17 **Walk** at a faster pace *for 15 mins*
WEEK 4	Day 22 **Walk** at a faster pace *for 25 mins*	Day 23 **Walk** at a faster pace *for 15 mins*	Day 24 **Walk** at a faster pace *for 20 mins*

Other pages to help you

• Walking to lose weight, see pp98–99 • Using a pedometer, see pp36–37 • Using a heart-rate monitor, see pp36–37 • Hill walking, see pp112–113 • Any other activity, see pp134–137 • Think positive, see pp78–79 • Posture and breathing, see pp40–41 • Foods for fitness, see pp90–91

Use this program as a guide and adapt it to suit your life. Take into account your weight and fitness to determine which week of the program you should start at. Your goal is to achieve a good pace and to maintain it for an hour. As you progress, you will find that you are able to walk farther in the same amount of time. Start at a pace that is a little faster than your normal pace and increase the distance and speed as you feel ready. If your body is not used to exercise, it will need a bit of a push each time you walk, but persevere. Try never to miss more than one day of the program in any given week.

Key

Walk days

Other activity days

Rest days

WEDNESDAY	THURSDAY	FRIDAY	SATURDAY	
Day 4	**Day 5**	**Day 6**	**Day 7**	**Total**
Walk at a steady pace *for 10 mins*	**Walk** at a steady pace *for 10 mins*	**Walk** at a steady pace *for 15 mins*	**Walk** at a steady pace *for 10 mins*	**75 mins**
Day 11	**Day 12**	**Day 13**	**Day 14**	**Total**
Walk at a steady pace *for 10 mins*	**Walk** at a steady pace *for 15 mins*	**Walk** at a steady pace *for 10 mins*	**Walk** at a steady pace *for 15 mins*	**90 mins**
Day 18	**Day 19**	**Day 20**	**Day 21**	**Total**
Walk at a faster pace *for 20 mins*	**Walk** at a faster pace *for 15 mins*	**Walk** at a faster pace *for 15 mins*	**Walk** at a faster pace *for 20 mins*	**120 mins**
Day 25	**Day 26**	**Day 27**	**Day 28**	**Total**
Walk at a faster pace *for 25 mins*	**Walk** at a faster pace *for 15 mins* + *any other activity for 20 mins*	**Walk** at a faster pace *for 20 mins*	**Walk** at a faster pace *for 20 mins*	**140 mins**

Exercise pages
• Warming up and cooling down, see Warm-up and cooldown plan p72   • Stretch and strengthen, see Stretching and strengthening plan p73

WEIGHT LOSS: STAGE 2

Weeks 5–8

By now you will have a routine in place and be developing your favorite walks. You should also be able to walk farther in the same amount of time.

It is a good idea to introduce a different activity to your training plan now. This can be anything that will again increase your heart rate, such as swimming or dancing. Most importantly, it must be accessible and you must enjoy it.

You also have the option to include hill walking in these weeks. This means finding a route with hills, or using a treadmill on a minimum incline of 2. By walking on hills, you will be working your body harder and burning more energy. If you do not yet feel ready for this, you can include this into your plan a bit later, at any time you choose.

	SUNDAY	**MONDAY**	**TUESDAY**
WEEK 5	Day 29 **Walk** at a faster pace *for 30 mins*	Day 30 **Walk** at a faster pace *for 20 mins*	Day 31 **Walk** at a faster pace *for 25 mins*
WEEK 6	Day 36 **Walk** at a faster pace *for 25 mins*	Day 37 **Walk** at a faster pace *for 30 mins* *+ any other activity* *for 30 mins*	Day 38 **Walk** at a faster pace *for 20 mins*
WEEK 7	Day 43 **Walk** at a faster pace *for 35 mins*	Day 44 **Walk** at a faster pace *for 20 mins*	Day 45 **Walk** at a faster pace *for 35 mins*
WEEK 8	Day 50 **Walk** at a faster pace *for 40 mins*	Day 51 **Walk** at a faster pace *for 30 mins*	Day 52 **Walk** at a faster pace *for 20 mins*

Other pages to help you
• Walking to lose weight, see pp98–99 • Using a pedometer, see pp36–37 • Using a heart-rate monitor, see pp36–37 • Hill walking, see pp112–113 • Any other activity, see pp134–137 • Think positive, see pp78–79 • Posture and breathing, see pp40–41 • Foods for fitness, see pp90–91

WEDNESDAY	**THURSDAY**	**FRIDAY**	**SATURDAY**	
Day 32	Day 33	Day 34	Day 35	Total
Walk at a faster pace *for 30 mins*	**Walk** at a faster pace *for 30 mins*	**Walk** at a faster pace *for 25 mins* *+ any other activity* *for 15–20 mins*	**Walk** at a faster pace *for 30 mins*	190 mins
Day 39	Day 40	Day 41	Day 42	Total
Walk at a faster pace *for 30 mins*	**Walk** at a faster pace *for 20 mins*	**Walk** at a faster pace *for 20 mins*	**Walk** at a faster pace *for 30 mins*	175 mins
Day 46	Day 47	Day 48	Day 49	Total
Walk at a faster pace *for 20 mins* *+ any other activity* *for 30 mins*	**Walk** at a faster pace *for 35 mins*	**Hill walking** at a faster pace *for 20 mins*	**Walk** at a faster pace *for 35 mins*	200 mins
Day 53	Day 54	Day 55	Day 56	Total
Walk at a faster pace *for 40 mins*	**Walk** at a faster pace *for 30 mins*	**Walk** at a faster pace *for 20 mins*	**Walk** at a faster pace *for 20 mins* *+ any other activity* *for 30 mins*	200 mins

Key

Walk days

Other activity days

Rest days

Exercise pages
• Warming up and cooling down, see Warm-up and cooldown plan p72 • Stretch and strengthen, see Stretching and strengthening plan p73

WEIGHT LOSS: STAGE 3

Weeks 9–12

These final weeks of the training plan are all at speed. This means that by now you should be able to push yourself and reach a 14–16-minute pace per 1 mile (1.6km).

At this point, you can challenge yourself to cover different terrain, collecting a repertoire of walks that will keep you motivated to keep going. Reaching 12 weeks is a great achievement, so well done to you!

You can of course keep walking and continue the pattern of walking for the same time, but continually aim to increasing your speed and distance within that time. This is a great way to increase your fitness. Or you could feel you are ready to take on a challenge, such as a half-marathon. Whatever you choose, by continuing to walk and by eating healthier foods, there is every chance that you can maintain your ideal weight.

You may also want to start walking toward the magical 10,000 steps a day. If you have a sedentary job, you may be very surprised at how few steps you are taking outside of this training plan. Aim to use your daily walk as part of your 10,000 steps and watch the difference that being more mobile makes to every aspect of your life.

Try gathering together a group of like-minded people with a similar goal as yourself. Walking with others is not only sociable and fun, but there is also always motivation and support on hand whenever you need it.

	SUNDAY	**MONDAY**	**TUESDAY**
WEEK 9	Day 57 **Walk** at speed *for 40 mins*	Day 58 **Walk** at speed *for 45 mins*	Day 59 **Walk** at speed *for 30 mins* *+ any other activity* *for 30 mins*
WEEK 10	Day 64 **Walk** at speed *for 45 mins*	Day 65 **Walk** at speed *for 35 mins*	Day 66 **Walk** at speed *for 45 mins*
WEEK 11	Day 71 **Walk** at speed *for 35 mins*	Day 72 **Walk** at speed *for 50 mins* *+ any other activity* *for 30 mins*	Day 73 **Walk** at speed *for 35 mins*
WEEK 12	Day 78 **Walk** at speed *for 40 mins*	Day 79 **Walk** at speed *for 45 mins*	Day 80 **Walk** at speed *for 50 mins*

Other pages to help you
• Walking to lose weight, see pp98–99 • Using a pedometer, see pp36–37 • Using a heart-rate monitor, see pp36–37 • Hill walking, see pp112–113 • Any other activity, see pp134–137 • Think positive, see pp78–79 • Posture and breathing, see pp40–41 • Foods for fitness, see pp90–91

WEDNESDAY	THURSDAY	FRIDAY	SATURDAY	
Day 60 **Walk** at speed *for 45 mins*	Day 61 **Walk** at speed *for 30 mins*	Day 62 **Walk** at speed *for 45 mins*	Day 63 **Walk** at speed *for 30 mins*	Total **265 mins**
Day 67 **Walk** at speed *for 45 mins*	Day 68 **Walk** at speed *for 45 mins* *+ any other activity* *for 30 mins*	Day 69 **Walk** at speed *for 35 mins*	Day 70 **Walk** at speed *for 45 mins*	Total **295 mins**
Day 74 **Walk** at speed *for 35 mins*	Day 75 **Walk** at speed *for 35 mins*	Day 76 **Walk** at speed *for 45 mins*	Day 77 **Walk** at speed *for 50 mins*	Total **285 mins**
Day 81 **Walk** at speed *for 45 mins*	Day 82 **Walk** at speed *for 50 mins*	Day 83 **Walk** at speed *for 45 mins* *+ any other activity* *for 30 mins*	Day 84 **Walk** at speed *for 60 mins*	Total **335 mins**

Exercise pages
• Warming up and cooling down, see Warm-up and cooldown plan p72 • Stretch and strengthen, see Stretching and strengthening plan p73

Key

Walk days

Other activity days

Rest days

EXTREME: STAGE 1

The intensity of training to reach the required fitness level for an extreme challenge of any distance demands dedicated commitment. You will be placing a significant demand for both an increase of your time and physical effort. But, if you prepare, the reward is thrilling and definitely worth reaching for.

It is worth noting that for those wanting to achieve the required starting fitness, or for those taking on 100km challenge or back-to-back consecutive marathons, it is advisable to add a further 4 weeks onto your training plan to allow more time to reach your peak. Also consider a longer pre-event walk if you are walking further than 26 miles (42km). With any intense training, it is important to always be aware of how you feel. If at any point you feel uncomfortable or unwell, consult medical advice immediately.

Weeks 1–4

Use the time over the next 4 weeks to get into a routine. Finding the space in your life to fit in the miles and activities can be as challenging as actually doing them. Once you have a schedule, book it into your diary as appointments so that you are less likely to change them.

You will notice that the plan has been designed to follow a week-by-week schedule, completing certain activities on the same day each week. The order can be changed to fit into your life as long as the total sessions each week are the same.

These first weeks are also an important time to try out different activities. If you are a member of a gym, book an assessment with a trainer so that he can put a program together for you using cross training equipment. Although you do not have to stick to the same activities throughout, it does help initially to create a routine. There is a lot to think about, so the more it can be streamlined to get going the better.

	SUNDAY	MONDAY	TUESDAY
WEEK 1	**Day 1** **Walk 5 miles** (8km) *and stretch*	**Day 2** **Rest** *and stretch*	**Day 3** **Cross training or any other activity** *30–45 mins* Try something new!
WEEK 2	**Day 8** **Walk 6 miles** (9.6km) *and stretch*	**Day 9** **Rest** *and stretch*	**Day 10** **Cross training or any other activity** *30–45 mins* Try Pilates or kettlebell
WEEK 3	**Day 15** **Walk 8 miles** (12.9km) *and stretch*	**Day 16** **Rest** *and stretch*	**Day 17** **Cross training or any other activity** *30–45 mins* Try 15 mins of swimming or Pilates after
WEEK 4	**Day 22** **Walk 10 miles** (16km) *and stretch*	**Day 23** **Rest** *and stretch*	**Day 24** **Cross training or any other activity** *45 mins*

Other pages to help you

• Foods for fitness pp90–91 • Preparing for a marathon, see pp106–107 • Any other activity, see pp134–137 • Interval training, see pp110–111 • Meeting the challenge pp80–81

The overall aim of this plan is to build total body strength, stamina, and fitness for those wanting to complete an extreme marathon distance, a longer distance, or trek. To begin this plan assumes you have a good level of basic fitness and walking ability. You must be able to comfortably walk 4 miles (6.5km) consecutively at a 14–15 minute per mile (1.6km) pace. Emphasis is also put onto cross training and other activities in order to help you develop the overall strength that is required to meet an extreme or ultra challenge. If you are uncertain about your starting fitness, turn to pages 170–171 and complete the first 4 weeks of the Marathon program before beginning the Extreme program.

Key
- Walk days
- Other activity days
- Rest days

WEDNESDAY	THURSDAY	FRIDAY	SATURDAY	
Day 4 **Walk 5 miles** (8km) *and stretch*	**Day 5** **Rest** *and stretch*	**Day 6** **Walk 5 miles** (8km) *and stretch*	**Day 7** **Swim** *30 mins*	**Total** **15 miles** (24km)
Day 11 **Walk 6 miles** (9.6km) *and stretch*	**Day 12** **Rest** *and stretch*	**Day 13** **Walk 6 miles** (9.6km) *and stretch*	**Day 14** **Swim** *30 mins*	**Total** **18 miles** (28.2km)
Day 18 **Walk 6 miles** (9.6km) *and stretch* Try some hills or an incline on a treadmill	**Day 19** **Rest** *and stretch*	**Day 20** **Walk 6 miles** (9.6km) *and stretch*	**Day 21** **Swim** *30 mins*	**Total** **20 miles** (32km)
Day 25 **Walk 6 miles** (9.6km) *and stretch* Don't forget to choose different routes!	**Day 26** **Rest** *and stretch*	**Day 27** **Walk 8 miles** (12.9km) *and stretch*	**Day 28** **Swim** *40 mins*	**Total** **24 miles** (38.6km)

Exercise Pages
- Stretching exercises pp60–67 • Warming up and cooling down, see Warm-up and Cool-down sequences p72 • Swimming and Kettlebells, see pp134–135

EXTREME: STAGE 2

Weeks 5–6

Over the next 2 weeks the miles begin to increase and you should now be in the swing of it. Use this time to work on your technique—it will be impossible to reach your goal without using good technique. Work on streamlining your body and using your arms to their full potential to propel you forward.

Do not make the common mistake of skipping the stretches, either before, during, or after your walks, or on your rest days. The power of stretching can only be discovered if you actually commit to doing them properly, but once you do, you will never look back!

You may want to consider using 2 pairs of shoes to alternate for training so that if it rains you always have dry shoes.

Weeks 7–8

Support your body by eating well. You will probably find your appetite increases quite considerably. Always make sure you have some healthy snacks on hand and good food in the fridge. The temptation is to eat whatever you can put your hands on first, so make sure it's not junk.

You will be out walking for many hours, so being hydrated is an important part of your preparation. Poor hydration will not help your form on the day. Many people start drinking a lot of water on the day of the challenge, which is not only unnecessary, but uncomfortable, and it usually means you spend a lot of wasted time queuing for restrooms. Drinking more water and being hydrated should start in the early stages of training. It takes your body some time to become used to extra liquid; however, persist and your body will reward you by helping you to be in the best shape you can on the day of the event.

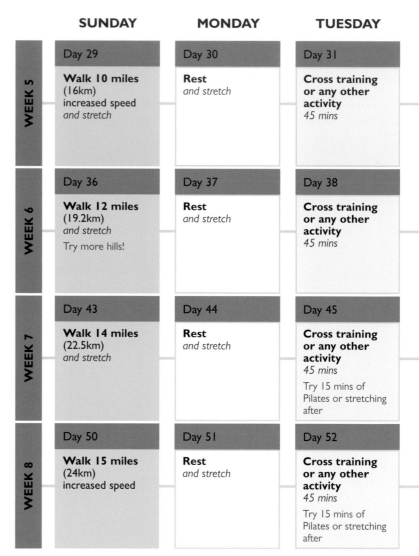

	SUNDAY	MONDAY	TUESDAY
WEEK 5	Day 29 **Walk 10 miles (16km)** increased speed *and stretch*	Day 30 **Rest** *and stretch*	Day 31 **Cross training or any other activity** *45 mins*
WEEK 6	Day 36 **Walk 12 miles (19.2km)** *and stretch* Try more hills!	Day 37 **Rest** *and stretch*	Day 38 **Cross training or any other activity** *45 mins*
WEEK 7	Day 43 **Walk 14 miles (22.5km)** *and stretch*	Day 44 **Rest** *and stretch*	Day 45 **Cross training or any other activity** *45 mins* Try 15 mins of Pilates or stretching after
WEEK 8	Day 50 **Walk 15 miles (24km)** increased speed	Day 51 **Rest** *and stretch*	Day 52 **Cross training or any other activity** *45 mins* Try 15 mins of Pilates or stretching after

Other pages to help you
• Foods for fitness pp90–91 • Preparing for a marathon, see pp106–107 • Any other activity, see pp134–137 • Interval training, see pp110–111 • Meeting the challenge pp80–81

WEDNESDAY	THURSDAY	FRIDAY	SATURDAY	
Day 32	**Day 33**	**Day 34**	**Day 35**	Total
Walk 6 miles (9.6km) *and stretch* Try interval training for 20 mins of your walk	**Rest** *and stretch*	**Walk 8 miles** (12.9km) *and stretch*	**Swim** *40 mins + 15 mins stretching*	**24 miles** (38.6km)
Day 39	**Day 40**	**Day 41**	**Day 42**	Total
Walk 8 miles (12.9km) *and stretch* Try interval training for 20 mins of your walk	**Rest** *and stretch*	**Walk 10 miles** (16km) *and stretch*	**Swim** *40 mins + 15 mins stretching*	**30 miles** (48km)
Day 46	**Day 47**	**Day 48**	**Day 49**	Total
Walk 8 miles (12.9km) picking up the pace *and stretch*	**Rest** *and stretch*	**Walk 10 miles** (16km) *and stretch*	**Swim** *45 mins + 15 mins stretching*	**32 miles** (51.4km)
Day 53	**Day 54**	**Day 55**	**Day 56**	Total
Walk 10 miles (16km) *and stretch*	**Rest** *and stretch*	**Walk 10 miles** (16km) *and stretch*	**Swim** *45 mins + 15 mins stretching*	**35 miles** (56km)

Key

Walk days

Other activity days

Rest days

Exercise Pages
• Stretching exercises pp60–67 • Warming up and cooling down, see Warm-up and Cool-down sequences p72 • Swimming and Kettlebells, see pp134–135

EXTREME: STAGE 3

Weeks 9–12

Don't forget to alternate and change your route regularly so that it is fresh and interesting.

Two weeks in advance of your challenge you will reach your climax in training.

By now you should feel powerful and strong as you walk. Whatever your challenge, completing this distance or longer is an important step to mentally and physically give you the confidence to achieve your goal.

It will take your body approximately 2 weeks to recover from the long walk, so help it along with plenty of good food, relaxation, stretching, and sleep.

Use visualization to see yourself crossing the finish line and receiving your medal. 65 percent of a challenge is mental so if you think you can you will, and if you think you can't you won't!

	SUNDAY	MONDAY	TUESDAY
WEEK 9	Day 57 **Walk 16 miles (25.7km)** *and stretch*	Day 58 **Rest** *and stretch*	Day 59 **Cross training or any other activity** *45 mins*
WEEK 10	Day 64 **Walk 18 miles (29km)** *and stretch*	Day 65 **Rest** *and stretch*	Day 66 **Cross training or any other activity** *45 mins*
WEEK 11	Day 71 **Walk 20 miles (32km)**	Day 72 **Rest** *and stretch*	Day 73 **Swim** *30 mins*
WEEK 12	Day 78 **Walk 7 miles (11.2km)** *and stretch*	Day 79 **Rest** *and stretch*	Day 80 **Rest** *and stretch*
WEEK 13	Day 85 **Challenge Day**	**Well Done!**	

WEDNESDAY	THURSDAY	FRIDAY	SATURDAY	
Day 60 **Walk 10 miles** (16km) *and stretch*	**Day 61** **Rest** *and stretch*	**Day 62** **Walk 12 miles** (19.3km) *and stretch*	**Day 63** **Swim** *45 mins*	**Total** **38 miles** (61km)
Day 67 **Walk 10 miles** (16km) at speed *and stretch*	**Day 68** **Rest** *and stretch*	**Day 69** **Walk 14 miles** (22.5km) *and stretch*	**Day 70** **Swim** *45 mins*	**Total** **42 miles** (67.5km)
Day 74 **Rest** *and stretch*	**Day 75** **Walk 8 miles** (12.9km) *and stretch*	**Day 76** **Cross training or any other activity**	**Day 77** **Swim** *30 mins*	**Total** **28 miles** (44.9km)
Day 81 **Walk 5 miles** (8km) *and stretch*	**Day 82** **Swim** *45 mins*	**Day 83** **Rest** *and stretch*	**Day 84** **Walk 5 miles** (8km) *and stretch*	**Total** **17 miles** (27.2km)

Key

- Walk days
- Other activity days
- Rest days

Exercise Pages
- Stretching exercises pp60–67 • Warming up and cooling down, see Warm-up and Cool-down sequences p72 • Swimming and Kettlebells, see pp134–135

USEFUL RESOURCES

American Podiatric Medical Association
Tel: (800) ASK-APMA
www.apma.org
For details of qualified local practitioners.

Canadian Podiatric Medical Association
Tel: (800) 220-3338
www.podiatrycanada.org
For details of local Canadian practitioners.

TheraGear, Inc.
Tel: (888) 474-7735
www.theragear.com
For exercise balls.

Reebok International Ltd.
Tel: (866) 271-5859
www.reebok.com
Manufacturer of good walk-specific shoes.

Polar Electro Inc.
Tel: (800) 227-1314
www.polar.com
For heart-rate monitors and related products.

American Volkssport Association
Tel: (800) 830-WALK
www.ava.org
Sponsors noncompetitive walking events across the nation.

American Discovery Trail
Tel: (800) 663-2387
www.discoverytrail.org
Manages the nation's only coast-to-coast, nonmotorized recreational trail.

America WALKS
Tel: (503) 222-1077
www.americawalks.org
National coalition promoting more walkable communities throughout America.

American Hiking Society
Tel: (301) 565-6704
www.americanhiking.org
National advocacy group; can help you get in contact with a hiking club in your area.

Orienteering USA
www.us.orienteering.org
For information on orienteering, and clubs and events in your area.

Walking to school
The following websites provide information and guidance for children and parents.
www.cdc.gov/nccdphp/dnpa/kidswalk
www.walkbiketoschool.org
www.safekidscanada.ca
www.goforgreen.ca

National Geographic Society
Tel: (800) 437-5521
www.nationalgeographic.com
Sells a wide variety of hiking and recreation maps.

Canadian Volkssport Federation
www.walks.ca
Organizes year-round noncompetitive walk events across Canada. Also provides links to clubs across the country.

Parks Canada
(888) 773-8888
www.pc.gc.ca
Provides a list of Canada's national parks.

Trans Canada Trail Association
Tel: (800) 465-3636
www.tctrail.ca
*The Trans Canada Trail makes its way through
every province and territory. The website provides
a detailed trail locator with more than 300 trails to
choose from, linking more than 750 cities and towns
across Canada.*

EPA, Office of Ground Water and Drinking Water
Tel: (202) 564-3750
www.epa.gov/safewater
Provides information on the safety of local tap water.

Walk the Walk Worldwide
United Kingdom
Tel: 01483 741430
www.walkthewalk.org
*For information on power walking, events worldwide
and how to join them, and lots more.*

Recommended reading

Any cookbooks by Jane Sen (Thorsons
Publishing Group)
*Beautiful books with easy-to-follow recipes and
practical advice.*

Bean, Anita, *Food for Fitness* (Hunter House, 2002)
A book specifically on sports nutrition.

INDEX

ACKNOWLEDGMENTS

Author's acknowledgments

This book has been created with the help and support of some very special people. I want to thank my partner, Guy, who modeled his walking skills and supported me with patience and a smile, for which I cannot thank him enough; my family for always believing in me; Sonia Doherty for her chiropractic skills and knowledge: Jane Sen for her wonderful attitude toward food; Nigel Fisher for his help with podiatry and chiropody; Cathy Orpin for her advice on Pilates; and Clare Maxwell-Hudson for her advice and encouragement.

I would also like to thank the team at DK, in particular my editors, Jennifer Lane and Jenny Jones, for their infinite patience and care, which I truly tested; Mary-Clare Jerram for recognizing just how important it was to have a book on power walking; and finally, to all my gorgeous, loving friends, who are always there for me!

A percentage of the royalties from this book will be donated to Walk the Walk Worldwide for breast cancer research and holistic cancer care.

Publisher's acknowledgments

Dorling Kindersley would like to thank photographer Russell Sadur and his assistant, Nina Duncan; models Guy Aubertin, Heidi Baillargeon, Lisa Rachel Bautista, Nikol Johnson, Cherie Greer, Amy Sobieraj, and Jennifer Lane; Sharon Weems for photo-shoot production and location services in Miami; clothes stylist Liz Hancock; Naomi @ Code Management for hair and makeup; art director Carol Ash; and Peter Rea for the index. Special thanks to Jo Lee at Reebok UK (www.reebok.co.uk) and Lynsey Mailer at Cake for all trainers provided; Leanne at USA Pro for sports clothing (www.usapro.co.uk); and www.heartratemonitor.co.uk for the heart-rate monitor.

Picture credits

The publisher would like to thank the following for their kind permission to reproduce their photographs: 36: iStockphoto.com: Franckreporter; 102: Masterfile UK/Ariel Skelley; 103: James Abelson; 104, 105, 189: courtesy of Walk the Walk Worldwide; 106: Empics Ltd; 113: Guy Aubertin. Illustrations by Phil Wilson. All other images © DK Images

About the author

Nina Barough has always been intrigued by the relationship and balance between the mind and body, and finds power walking a wonderful way of achieving this, while maintaining her passion for good health and fitness. She has been a vegetarian from a young age and has studied both massage and Reiki.

For many years, she ran her own successful production company. In 1996, her life changed when she had the idea of power walking the New York City Marathon wearing a customized bra in order to raise money and awareness for breast cancer causes. The idea became a reality, and the charity Walk the Walk was born.

Only months later, Nina was diagnosed with breast cancer, and her holistic knowledge and attitude toward health care played a vital part in her approach toward the treatment and recovery process. Walk the Walk Worldwide follows Nina's philosophy of life by encouraging people to take more responsibility for their well-being and to recognize their own potential for good health.

Nina was awarded a CBE in recognition of her charitable work. The charity organizes the annual MoonWalks held worldwide, and Nina continues to lead groups of power walkers in marathons and walking challenges around the world.